Make Health in India

Policy Studies Series

This series is designed to fill a visible gap in existing Social Sciences literature: the need to address, empirically investigate and rigorously analyse public policy in the field of governance.

It is important to study the policy world in its entirety because:

- Policies establish the context within which we live out our individual and collective lives and deeply impact the way we and future generations will live and work.
- Policy-making and implementation is a process that is deeply embedded in politics, and serves as an entry point into the politics of a country.
- Public administrators, scholars, journalists, and specialists need to understand the relationship between knowledge systems, technology and the making of policy, the nature of public participation and responses, and how politicians seek to forge networks to ensure that policy is transformed into law.
- Policy-making highlights the linkages between domestic and global contexts. Ideas disseminated through global institutions and civil society networks impact policy-making insofar as they influence identification of problems and propose resolutions.

The literature generated through the series, we hope, will serve to identify the strength and lacunae of the making of policy and its implementation in India.

Make Health in India

Reaching a Billion Plus

K. Srinath Reddy

Orient BlackSwan

MAKE HEALTH IN INDIA: REACHING A BILLION PLUS

ORIENT BLACKSWAN PRIVATE LIMITED

Registered Office
3-6-752 Himayatnagar, Hyderabad 500 029, Telangana, India
e-mail: centraloffice@orientblackswan.com

Other Offices
Bengaluru, Chennai, Guwahati, Hyderabad,
Kolkata, Mumbai, New Delhi, Noida, Patna

First published by Orient BlackSwan in 2019
Reprinted 2020, 2024

040968

ISBN 978-93-5287-678-5

Typeset in
ITC Berkeley Oldstyle Std 10.5/14
by Le Studio Graphique, Gurgaon 122 001

Printed in India at
Avantika Printers Private Limited, New Delhi 110 020

Published by
Orient BlackSwan Private Limited
3-6-752 Himayatnagar, Hyderabad 500 029, Telangana, India
e-mail: info@orientblackswan.com

To the memories of
my father, K. V. Raghunatha Reddy, who gave me
the dream of a just and equitable society,
and my mother, C. Sarojini Reddy,
who reflected it in the reality of committed,
competent and compassionate healthcare.

Contents

Figures and Tables

Figures

Tables

Abbreviations

ANM	Auxiliary Nurse Midwives
ASHA	Accredited Social Health Activist
AYUSH	Ayurveda, Yoga, Unani, Siddha and Homeopathy
BRHC	Bachelor of Rural Health Care
CPHC	Comprehensive Primary Health Care
CVD	cardiovascular disease
DALY	Disability Adjusted Life Year
EAG	Empowered Action Group
FTA	Free Trade Agreement
GDP	gross domestic product
HLEG	High Level Expert Group
HWC	Health and Wellness Centre
IMA	Indian Medical Association
IMR	infant mortality rate
ISDS	Investor State Dispute Settlement
MCI	Medical Council of India
MDG	Millennium Development Goals
MPPEB	Madhya Pradesh Professional Examination Board
NCD	non-communicable disease
NCHRH	National Commission on Human Resources in Health

NDRDA	National Drug Regulatory and Development Authority
NGO	non-governmental organisation
NHA	National Health Agency
NHM	National Health Mission
NHP	National Health Policy
NHPPT	National Health Promotion and Protective Trust
NHPS	National Health Protection Scheme
NHRDA	National Health Regulatory and Development Authority
NITI	National Institution for Transforming India
NLEM	National List of Essential Medicines
NMC	National Medical Commission
NRHM	National Rural Health Mission
OOPS	out-of-pocket spending
PHC	Primary Health Centre
PMJAY	Pradhan Mantri Jan Arogya Yojana
PPP	public–private partnership
RSBY	Rashtriya Swasthya Bima Yojana
SDG	sustainable development goals
SECC	Socio Economic and Caste Census
SHA	State Health Agency
SHRDA	State Health Regulatory and Development Authority
TRIPS	Trade Related Intellectual Property Rights
UHC	universal health coverage
VGF	Viability Gap Funding
WHO	World Health Organization
WTO	World Trade Organization

Preface

By 2025, India will be the most populous nation in the world. It is also poised to become the world's third largest economy by 2030. However, the health indicators of this large country lag behind its economic growth and compare poorly with those of most neighbours and peers. Beyond the aggregate national health indicators of concern, there is evidence of huge health inequalities across regional, urban–rural, socio-economic, gender, religious and caste strata. These pose a major threat to India's development and stability. There is an urgent need to steer our health policy to quickly gain ground in improving the health of our population and strengthen our health system to bridge the glaring gaps in health equity.

This book is an attempt to introduce issues related to India's health policy and health system to all Indians who are interested in paving India's path to sustainable and equitable development. It is not a book that aims to attract the attention of scholars and researchers. The intended readership is one of socially conscious citizens, be they from the circle of policymakers, civil society or media. I hope it will also engage the attention of the students of public health and set off debates among them. Health system managers, researchers, public health practitioners, healthcare providers and advocates who are actively engaged as change-makers for health-system transformation may not all agree with the perspectives or recommendations that are presented in the book. Nevertheless, I do hope it will stimulate energetic discussion that will position health centrally in public discourse.

Health, at both the population and individual levels, is influenced by many determinants. Several of them lie outside the conventional remit of health policy and services. From agriculture and food systems, urban design and transport, from education to employment, from environment to social stability, from gender to caste and social status—many influences coalesce to enable or erode the health of persons (individuals), people (communities) and populations (nations). To deal with these social, economic and environmental determinants of health is beyond the scope of this book, vital as they are. This book, therefore, is a modest attempt to portray the meandering path our health policy has followed over the past 15 years to increase the outreach, effectiveness and equity dimensions of India's health services. With the goal of achieving universal health coverage by 2030 challenging us, where have we reached in that journey and how do we proceed further? As a national election year, 2019 is perhaps the best time to engage political parties and citizens alike to take a fresh look at our health policy and needed reforms.

Policy will respond appropriately to India's health challenges only when citizens recognise that health is critical to development and that the many determinants of health need to be influenced to protect, preserve and promote the health at both the population and individual levels. A citizen movement is very much needed for advancing universal health coverage and multi-sectoral actions for health promotion, from aspirations to achieved objectives. Many sections of society, from all across the country, must partner to create such a movement and indicate the right direction to health policy and impart the required momentum to health transformation. This book is a humble offering to assist such a movement as it develops.

K. SRINATH REDDY
January 2019, New Delhi

Acknowledgements

A book lies dormant in the mind even as the desire to write flickers often, till a strong stimulus kindles the commitment to go ahead with the required discipline. For me, such a stimulus came from two sources. Ram Manohar Reddy, the Series Editor, contacted me to enquire if I would write a book on India's health policy. Around that time, my wife, Sunanda, too, was urging me to write a book that compiles my views on the health system and health policy in India. She was particularly concerned that the contribution of the High Level Expert Group (HLEG) to the discourse on Universal Health Coverage (UHC) in India was inadequately documented and likely to remain hidden from the citizens of this country, who have to ultimately drive informed choices in health policy. She argued that op-eds, which I used as my main channel of public communication, are like shooting stars that fade fast from vision and memory. Ram's invitation came at that opportune moment when the layers of procrastination that were wrapped around my desire to write were being stripped away by Sunanda. The big-banner announcement of Ayushman Bharat that followed the National Health Policy of 2017 also enlivened the public debates on health. A good time to write. Thank you, Ram and Sunanda, for nudging me to move from musings to manuscript.

I am highly indebted to Manu Mathur, my colleague at the Public Health Foundation of India (PHFI), who helped me with fact checks and referencing. My secretary, Aji Chellappan, was an ever dependable protector of the drafts which I mailed to him at odd times after composing them on my iPhone (my only writing instrument). I also express my sincere gratitude to Manu and Aji, who have given me invaluable support in composing and completing this book. I have learnt much on access to drugs from a senior PHFI colleague, Sakthivel Selvaraj, and gratefully acknowledge his help.

A major chapter in this book covers the report of the HLEG on UHC, constituted by the Planning Commission of India. While I had the privilege of chairing that group, the report represents the collective work of all the highly accomplished members the HLEG, who brought vast riches of expertise, experience, vision and values to the endeavour. I am beholden to these colleagues in the HLEG: A. K. Shiva Kumar, Gita Sen, Abhay Bang, Vinod Paul, Mirai Chatterjee, Amarjit Sinha, Nachiket Mor, Jasodhara Dasgupta, Leila Caleb Varkey, Yogesh Jain, N. K. Sethi, Govinda Rao, P. K. Pradhan and Anu Garg. Several technical experts of the PHFI also contributed to the development of the HLEG report, as part of the secretariat. It is time to thank them again.

The lively debates around health policy and UHC draw ideas and perspectives from many public health researchers and practitioners, civil society advocates, public-spirited civil servants, economists, clinicians from public and private sectors, and the media. I have been educated by their views and influenced by their critiques, even when there have been divergent opinions on some issues. I owe all of them thanks for shaping my views and look forward to their energetic exchanges, and even critical contestation on the contents of this book. From my friends in the civil society, I miss the electrifying presence of Amit Sengupta, whose incisive intellect and uncompromising defence of public interest will be an enduring inspiration even after his untimely demise.

The art of converting a manuscript into a book lies in the hands of the publisher. I am most grateful to Orient BlackSwan for publishing the book, and especially indebted to Parvati Mohan for devoting her time and talent to editorially review the manuscript with the greatest of care to correct its flaws. I could not have hoped for more meticulous attention and immensely helpful suggestions.

Finally, dear reader, I thank you for picking up this book, because it was to seek your attention to India's health that I have written it. We may not have met, but the hope that you will help to improve India's health has been my inspiration.

K. Srinath Reddy
February 2019

one

What Makes a Healthy Society?

'Health leaps out of science and draws nourishment from the totality of society.'

Gunnar Myrdal
(Swedish Nobel Laureate in Economics, 1974)

Health is often viewed as an individual attribute, to be enjoyed, tended to and mended at a personal level. This perspective imposes the responsibility of ill health on the individual and also heaps the physical, financial and emotional burdens of obtaining healthcare on that person. The role of a society's economic, social and political systems in shaping the health of the population and impacting an individual's health is unsighted in such a blinkered view.

Scientific knowledge does provide insights into the interplay of biology, beliefs and behaviours that operate at the individual level to determine the balance between health and illness at any stage of life. Indeed, the explosion of such scientific information is fascinating—whether it is the role of genetic influences, the huge microbial population that cohabits our bodies and influences our health, the effects of the living habits and physical environment that modify gene expression (epigenetic pathways of 'up' or 'down' regulation) or how our diet, activity and sleep patterns influence our hormones and the nervous system (Ursell, Metcalf, Parfrey and Knight 2012). However, these personal attributes, too, are significantly impacted by factors that operate at the family and community levels. They include perceptions of health that are culturally determined or shaped by media and marketing. Priorities at the household level may steer the finite financial resources towards the purchase of healthy foods or squandering a large part on tobacco and alcohol. Gender bias in feeding or seeking healthcare is another obvious manifestation of prejudiced priorities at the household level. Sacrificing a green space available for common recreation and physical activity for a commercial centre or ignoring the dangers of pollution from uncontrolled vehicular density and coal-based power plants represent skewed priorities at the community level. Pathways for accessing healthcare in the neighbourhood, securing tobacco- and smoke-free public spaces, green environments and safe pedestrian or cycling lanes on crowded roads are also factors that operate at the community level (Figure 1.1).

Figure 1.1: Cascade of Health Determinants

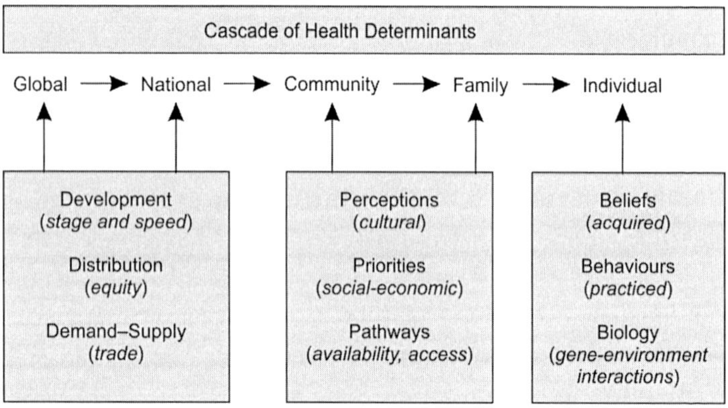

Source: Author.

Further upstream are the determinants that act at the national and global levels. They involve the level of economic development and the rate at which the economy is growing (Preston 1975). Of greater importance is how the fruits of that development are distributed across different sections of society, since inequality militates against a healthy society (Wilkinson and Pickett 2009). Such inequality manifests in many forms of active or passive discrimination, as society is stratified by income, gender, age, religion, caste and social status, but inevitably leads to poor health outcomes, whatever the form. At the global level, transnational trade and transport act as vectors of disease-causing agents like tobacco, and unhealthy foods and beverages, apart from pathogenic microbes (Kickbusch, Allen and Franz 2016). Trade also influences access to medicines, health technologies and availability of nutritious foods. The upstream determinants of health (economic, commercial and social) are increasingly influencing the health of populations and individuals (World Health Organization [WHO] 2008). While health policy, scripted by ministries of health, is usually confined to the services that the ministry is mandated to deliver, it has to necessarily take into account the bigger canvas of the varied influences that shape health through the cascade of multiple determinants.

Even when the perspective of the health policy is confined to the key elements of the health system that determine the nature of health services provided and the major social determinants of health, leaving aside complex areas like trade, the canvas is still large (Figure 1.2). The WHO listed six key elements of the health system, mainly from the perspective of a health ministry's mandate of designing, delivering and evaluating health services (WHO 2000). These are: infrastructure of healthcare facilities; the health workforce needed; availability of essential drugs and technologies; level and use of health financing; health information systems; and overall governance of the health services. It is natural that a health policy crafted by the health ministry deals with these elements in a detailed manner. A missing element in the WHO's list is the role of the community and its empowered engagement in the demand-driven design, delivery, monitoring and evaluation of health services. A national health policy can ill afford that omission.

Figure 1.2: Drivers of Health in Society

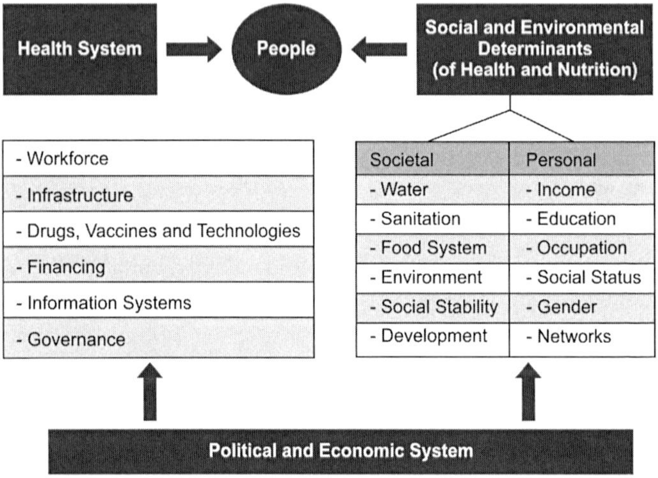

Source: Author.

It is at the level of the social determinants which shape health that health policy documents often tend to falter, with incomplete listing or superficial descriptions of intended approaches to influence them. The social determinants of health and nutrition that operate at the wider societal level include water, sanitation, the food system, physical environment, social stability and economic development. Those that operate at the individual level, although shaped by social forces, include income, education, occupation, social status, gender and participation in social networks.

Economic development and personal incomes exemplify the profound impact social determinants have on health. The economic growth of a country has a bi-directional relationship with the health of that population, with a prospering economy improving the health indicators and better health of the people, accelerating economic growth through increased productivity. Poverty has a bi-directional relationship with ill health at the personal level, with the poor more likely to become sick and less likely to access or afford healthcare, while ill health pushes persons into poverty because of lost wages and high cost of healthcare (Jamison, Summers, Aleyne, et al. 2013).

Equity becomes a very important factor when we examine how the nature of economic growth or social determinants influence the health of a population. The Preston Curve (Figure 1.3) illustrates how countries with low levels of per capita Gross Domestic Product (GDP) experience a sharp rise in life expectancy when that value rises, till an inflection point where that effect plateaus (Preston 1975). However, it has also been shown by Wilkinson and Pickett that income inequality within countries reduces the

Figure 1.3: Preston Curve

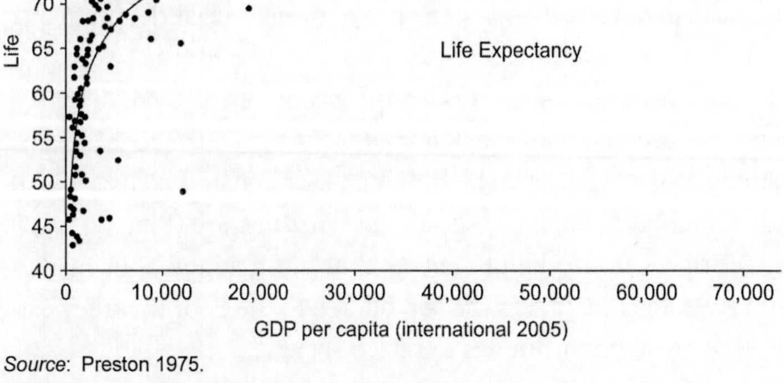

Source: Preston 1975.

benefit gained from economic growth (Wilkinson and Pickett 2006). At the same level of per capita GDP, countries with higher income inequality have lower life expectancy and worse health indicators than countries with lower levels of income inequality within their population.

Similarly, inequality in social determinants like education, nutrition, access to safe water, sanitation and clean energy affects the health of individuals even if health services are freely available to them. An undernourished child of uneducated parents from a poor family cannot grow as healthy as a child who is the well-nourished offspring of affluent and literate parents. Tragically, this effect can linger across several generations. If a pregnant woman is malnourished, not only will the female foetus in her womb be undernourished, but the ova of that baby, too, will experience epigenetic changes in gene expression that will manifest when that baby grows up to bear children. Both the child yet to be born and the child yet to be conceived become the victims of an intergenerational transmission of the effects of inequity (Reddy 2016).

The mere promise of universal health coverage and assured equality in access to health services will not correct these health effects of inequality in a society. Even if healthcare services provide equal access to the poor, the cumulative effects of multiple inequalities imposed on a person by adverse social determinants will damage health across the life course. In the words of an early twentieth-century British economist, R. H. Tawney, what is needed is 'an equal start, not just an open road'. In his book *Equality* (1924), which antedates Thomas Piketty's much acclaimed book *Capital in the Twenty-First Century* (Piketty 2013) by nearly a century, he presents a trenchant critique of inequality and scathingly dismisses the sop offered to the poor that they can avail of equal opportunities to rise in society:

> With massive inequalities, where many are denied an adequate education, unable to access effective health care and housed in slums, equality of opportunity is nothing more than a cruel jest—the impertinent courtesy of an invitation offered to unwelcome guests, in the certainty that circumstances will prevent them from accepting it (Tawney 1931).

Equity is often viewed as 'horizontal equity', which provides equal access to all for whatever services are on offer. If the carry-over effects of inequality are to be reduced, we also need to supplement it with 'vertical equity', where some additional services are preferentially provided to the disadvantaged and vulnerable sections of society to bridge the equity gaps in health and other social indicators. Both forms of equity require social solidarity, the former to do what is right and the latter to redress the wrong. Even in the context of Universal Health Coverage, where equal access is provided to all sections of society to a defined set of health services (horizontal equity), the poor and other vulnerable sections (such as the very young, elderly and disabled) would need specially targeted efforts to overcome disadvantages in access and affordability (vertical equity).

To minimise health inequalities in the first place, and to bridge health equity gaps when they do exist, the social determinants of health need to be addressed effectively in any efforts to build a healthy society. These determinants, and the way the health system is configured and managed to serve the needs of all sections of society, are ultimately dependant on the political and economic systems that steer society. Those who shape or interpret health policy should be cognisant of that, even if the policy is limited to the specific domain of the health sector. Even as health ministries configure national health policies mainly to improve health services, they must retain the ambition to study and influence the varied determinants of health that lie outside their conventional remit. A national health policy must project that holistic vision.

References

Commission on Social Determinants of Health. 2008. 'Closing the Gap in a Generation: Health Equity through Action on the Social Determinants of Health'. World Health Organization, Geneva.

Jamison, D. T., L. H. Summers, G. Alleyne, et al. 2013. 'Global Health 2035: A World Converging within a Generation'. *Lancet* 382 (9908): 1898–955.

Kickbusch, I., L. Allen, and C. Franz. 2016. 'The Commercial Determinants of Health'. *Lancet Global Health* 4 (12): PE895–PE896.

Piketty, T. 2013. *Capital in the Twenty-First Century*. Boston: Harvard University Press.

Preston, S. 1975. 'The Changing Relation between Mortality and Level of Economic Development'. *Population Studies (NY)* 29 (2): 231–48.

Reddy, K. S. 2016. 'Unequal by Birth: Time to Break the Vicious Cycle'. *The Hindu*, 7 March. Available at https://www.thehindu.com/opinion/op-ed/unequal-by-birth-time-to-break-the-vicious-cycle/article8320900.ece (accessed 8 December 2018).

Tawney, R. 1931. *Equality*. London: George Allen and Unwin.

Ursell, L., J. Metcalf, L. Parfrey, and R. Knight. 2012. 'Defining the Human Microbiome'. *Nutrition Reviews* 70 (1): S38–44.

Wilkinson, R. G., and K. Pickett. 2006. 'Income Inequality and Population Health: A Review and Explanation of the Evidence'. Social Science and Medicine 62 (7):1768–84.

———. 2009. *The Spirit Level: Why Greater Equality Makes Societies Stronger*. New York: Bloomsbury.

World Health Organization. 2000. 'The World Health Report 2000: Health Systems: Improving Performance', Geneva. Available at http://www.who.int/whr/2000/en/whr00_en.pdf (accessed 8 December 2018).

two

How Healthy is India?

> Do we not always find the diseases of the populace traceable to defects in society? ... If disease is an expression of individual life under unfavorable circumstances, then epidemics must be indicative of mass disturbances.
>
> Rudolf Virchow
> German Pathologist and Anthropologist (1821–1902)
> (DeWalt and Pincus 2003)

Health of a population is measured by key health indicators, which capture the impact of both social determinants and health system performance. Life expectancy at birth is a general measure that is often used. However, this does not tell how healthy those years were. Healthy life expectancy or healthy life years lost (in comparison to a standard population) is a measure that takes into account the years spent with disease. Disability Adjusted Life Year (DALY) is a measure that combines years of life lost due to a health condition (in comparison to an expected full life expectancy) and years lived with disability due to ill health (weighted for the degree of disability) (Abajobir, Abate, Abbafati, et al. 2017). Presently, it is a commonly used measure of disease burden caused by any or all diseases. More specific population level indicators that reflect specific health conditions are: infant mortality rate (IMR); neonatal mortality and under-5 child mortality (for child health); maternal mortality ratio (for childbirth-related deaths) and age-adjusted death rates for each disease.

Health status of a population does not remain static. It varies over time, as development lengthens life expectancy and replaces one dominant group of public health concerns with another. Health profile of populations across the world changes over time in response to socio-economic, demographic, nutritional, scientific, technological, environmental and cultural shifts (Rayner and Lang 2012). Such health transitions have been especially profound in the past half-century due to sweeping industrialisation, rapid urbanisation and relentless globalisation in most parts of the world. It is necessary to understand, and even predict, the patterns and dynamics of health transition so that multi-sectoral actions can be taken to protect and promote the health of populations.

Rayner and Lang describe nine transitions, which together shape the state of health in any population at a given time (Table 2.1).

Table 2.1: Transitions that Shape Public Health

Demographic	*Nutritional*	*Biological, Ecological*
Epidemiologic	Economic	Cultural
Urban	Energy	Democratic

Source: Adapted from Rayner and Lang 2012.

The pathway of health transition is conventionally seen as a shift from diseases of underdevelopment to disorders of maladapted modernity. The 'pre-transitional' disorders are a cluster of infectious and nutritional deficiency diseases, coupled with high maternal and child mortality, resulting in a low overall life expectancy. The post-transitional disorders are mostly non-communicable diseases (cardiovascular and chronic respiratory disorders, cancers and diabetes being the major ones), mental illness and injuries. However, health transition is not a simple linear process. The complexity introduced by distorted development and dysfunctional health systems may keep a population tethered to a high burden of 'pre-transitional' diseases despite obvious economic growth. Similarly, countries with strong political will to implement effective public policies directed at tobacco, unhealthy foods, pollution, and whose health systems are geared to early detection and control of chronic diseases can substantially limit the burden of the 'post-transitional' disorders even as they experience economic growth.

However, these transitions do not occur uniformly across a country, especially not in a large country like India. Different states, at varied levels of development, move at different speeds along the transition trajectory and, at any given time, present a different mix of public health challenges (Dandona, Dandona, Kumar, et al. 2017). Within each state, different profiles emerge across the rural–urban and rich–poor divides. In large states, sub-regional differences, too, will manifest, with the better-developed districts farther along in the transition path.

Life expectancy at birth improved in India from 59.7 years in 1990 to 70.3 years in 2016 for females, and from 58.3 years to 66.9 years for males. However, India's life expectancy has lagged behind many of its South Asian neighbours, despite having better economic growth (Figure 2.1). Moreover, life expectancy varies

Figure 2.1: Average Life Expectancy (Years) in 2015

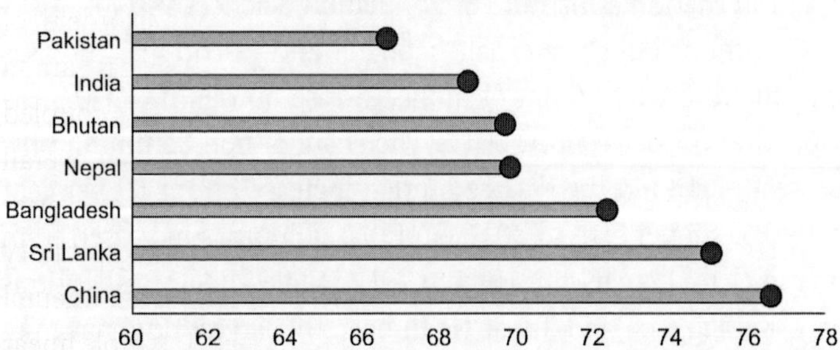

Source: Adapted by author from 'Universal Health Coverage (UHC) in India' (UHC Report 2018).

markedly between the states of India. Women in Uttar Pradesh have 12 years lower life expectancy than that of women in Kerala, while the life expectancy of men in Assam is 10 years lower than that of men in Kerala. The per-person disease burden from all causes dropped by 36 per cent in the same period. However, there was an almost two-fold difference between the states in 2016, with Assam, Uttar Pradesh and Chhattisgarh having the highest rates, and Kerala and Goa the lowest rates.

The under-5 mortality rate has reduced substantially in all states between 1990 and 2015. However, there was a four-fold difference in this rate between the highest, in Assam and Uttar Pradesh, as compared with the lowest, in Kerala in 2016 (Figure 2.2). Despite a decline from 1990 levels, child and maternal malnutrition remains the single largest risk factor, contributing to 15 per cent of the disease burden in 2016 (Figure 2.3). With its under-5 mortality six times higher than Sri Lanka and burden of child and maternal malnutrition 12 times higher than in China, India has wide gaps to bridge. Even when it comes to total immunisation rate in children, a sensitive indicator of health system performance, India has recorded a low coverage of 62–64 per cent, while many countries with much lower levels of economic development in South Asia and Sub-Saharan Africa have over 90 per cent coverage (Dandona, Dandona, Kumar, et al. 2017; International Institute of Population Sciences 2017).

Communicable, maternal, neonatal and nutritional diseases contributed to 61 per cent of India's disease burden in 1990. This dropped to 33 per cent in 2016. The share of non-communicable diseases (NCDs) in the disease burden increased from 30 per cent in 1990 to 55 per cent in 2016, and that of injuries increased from 9 per cent to 12 per cent (Figure 2.4). While all states show this trend, Kerala, Goa and Tamil Nadu have the largest dominance of NCDs and injuries over infectious and associated diseases, whereas

Figure 2.2: Under-5 Mortality Rate in the States of India

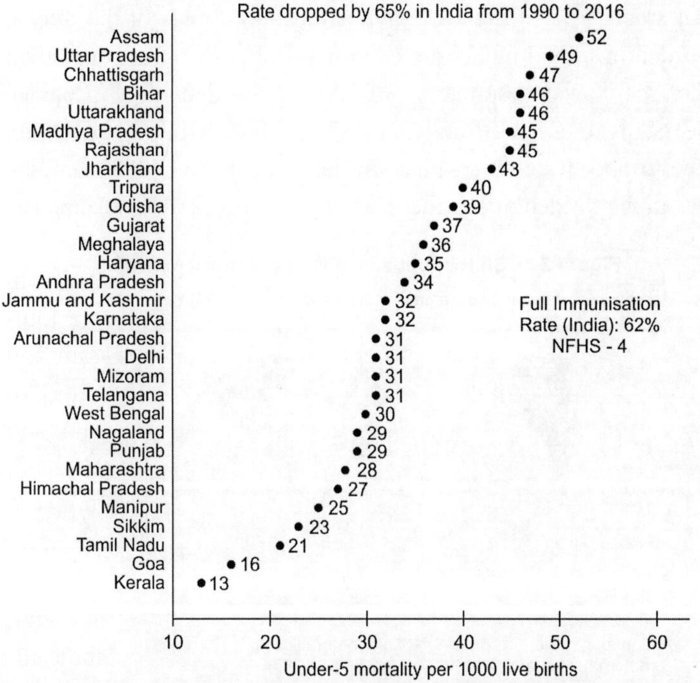

Under-5 mortality rate in India 5 times higher than in Sri Lanka and China in 2016

Source: Adapted by author from International Institute of Population Sciences 2017.

Figure 2.3: Trends in Nutritional Status in India, 1990–2016

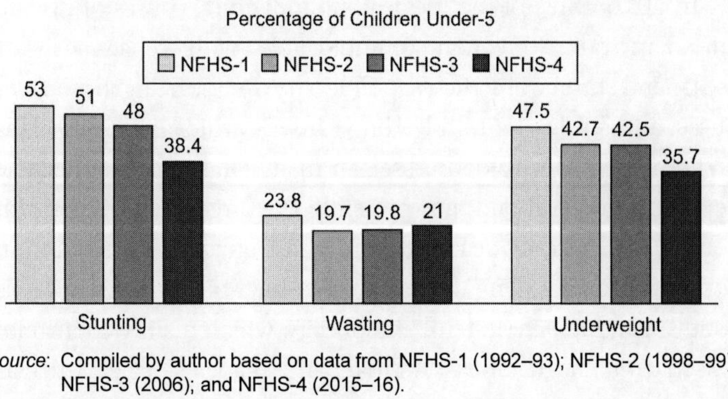

Source: Compiled by author based on data from NFHS-1 (1992–93); NFHS-2 (1998–99); NFHS-3 (2006); and NFHS-4 (2015–16).

this ratio is much lower in Bihar, Jharkhand, Uttar Pradesh and Rajasthan. Five of the 10 individual leading causes of the disease burden in India in 2016 are carry-overs of past threats: diarrhoeal diseases, lower respiratory infections, iron-deficiency anaemia, neonatal pre-term birth and tuberculosis. Though the disease burden due to poor water and sanitation decreased in these 25 years, the per capita burden due to these factors is 40 times that in China.

Figure 2.4: Shift in Causes of Disease Burden in India

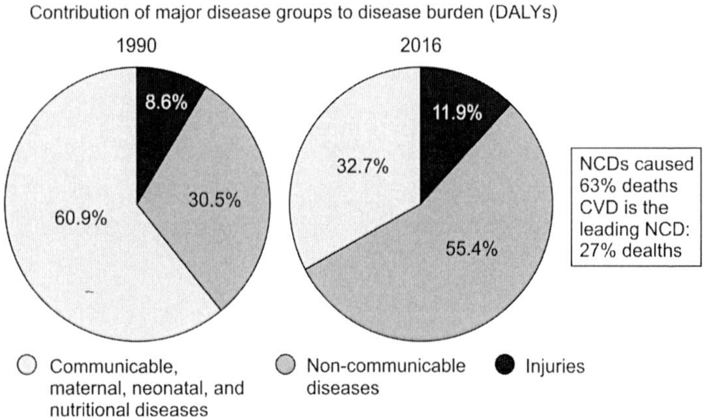

Source: Compiled by author on the basis of state-level disease burden in India study estimates.

In 2016, three of the five leading individual causes of disease burden in India were non-communicable, with ischaemic heart disease and chronic obstructive pulmonary disease being the top two causes, and stroke the fifth leading cause. Cardiovascular diseases (CVD), which affect blood vessels in many vital organs, especially the heart and the brain, are presently the largest contributors to mortality because of deaths due to heart attacks and strokes. A group of risks including unhealthy diet, high blood pressure, high blood sugar, high cholesterol and obesity, which mainly contribute to ischaemic heart disease, stroke and diabetes, caused about

25 per cent of the total disease burden in India in 2016, up from about 10 per cent in 1990. Ambient air pollution and household air pollution both rank high as risk factors in 2016, the former rising and the latter declining in the past 25 years (Dandona, Dandona, Kumar, et al. 2017). There were large variations between states in the degree to which these risks are rising. States in the early stages of the health transition were coping with both the persisting challenge of infectious, nutritional and pregnancy-related health threats, and the rising magnitude of NCDs. States in the advanced stage of the transition were grappling mostly with NCDs.

These data, of time trends and inter-state variations, highlight the need to develop specific strategies to address the major contributors to disease burden within each state. Disaggregated data, as provided in a recent report (Dandona, Dandona, Kumar, et al. 2017), will help to tailor customised state-level responses, while summated time trends will help the National Health Policy to set and track the progress towards country-level targets. Since the report provides modelled estimates derived from multiple and often limited datasets, it is imperative to strengthen vital registration mechanisms and strengthen disease and risk factor surveillance systems in every state. The broad national agenda should be elimination of malnutrition, reduction of child and maternal mortality, control of infectious diseases, and containment of risk factors contributing to NCDs. This report provides each state the GPS to chart its individual journey towards those goals, from different starting points.

India's health policy has to take note of the following facts:

1. Health transition is evident across the country, but with different states presently located at different stages. So, state-specific health policies are essential to address local priorities, even as the national policy provides a guiding framework.

2. On most health indicators, India's progress lags behind the levels anticipated from the country's economic growth. It is necessary to study to what extent inequalities resulting from non-inclusive growth, lack of attention to the social determinants of health and health system failures resulting from under-resourcing and poor governance have contributed to this. Unless correctives are applied across the board, health policy will not achieve its goals and time-bound targets.

References

Abajobir, A. A., K. H. Abate, C. Abbafati, et al. 2017. 'Global, Regional, and National Disability-Adjusted Life-Years (DALYs) for 333 Diseases and Injuries and Healthy Life Expectancy (HALE) for 195 Countries and Territories, 1990–2016: A Systematic Analysis for the Global Burden of Disease Study 2016'. *Lancet* 390 (10100): P1260–344.

Dandona, L., R. Dandona, G. A. Kumar, et al. 2017. 'Nations within a Nation: Variations in Epidemiological Transition across the States of India, 1990–2016 in the Global Burden of Disease Study'. *Lancet* 390 (10111): 2437–60.

DeWalt, D. A., and T. Pincus. 2003. 'The Legacies of Rudolf Virchow: Cellular Medicine in the 20th Century and Social Medicine in the 21st Century'. *Israel Medical Association Journal* 5 (6): 395–97.

International Institute of Population Sciences. 2017. 'National Family Health Survey 4; India Fact Sheet'. Ministry of Health and Family Welfare. Available at http://rchiips.org/NFHS/pdf/NFHS4/India.pdf (accessed 25 October 2018).

Rayner, G., and T. Lang. 2012. *Ecological Public Health: Reshaping the Conditions for Good Health*. Abingdon, UK: Routledge/Earthscan.

'Universal Health Coverage (UHC) in India: A Call for Greater Political Commitment and Public Financing'. 2018. Available at https://www.theelders.org/sites/default/files/the_elders_-_uhc_india_health_report_final-forweb_0.pdf (accessed 25 October 2018).

three

Health System Challenges

> The building blocks do not alone constitute a system, any more than a pile of bricks constitute a functioning building. It is the multiple relationships and interactions among the blocks—how one affects and influences the others, and is in turn affected by them—that converts these blocks into a system.
>
> de Savigny and Adam 2009

The WHO defines a health system as consisting of 'all organisations, people and actions whose primary interest is to promote, restore or maintain health'. It lists six building blocks as the components of the health system: leadership or governance; healthcare financing; health workforce; medical products and technologies; information and research; and service delivery (WHO 2000). Building on these, and promoting access, coverage, quality and safety, the health system is expected to assure improved health services (at different levels and with equity), responsiveness, financial risk protection and improved efficiency. Though community empowerment has not been explicitly mentioned as a building block, people will have to be at the centre of the health system. Community-centred public health and person-centred healthcare have to be the cardinal attributes of a caring health system.

India's health system has many mixes: state and central health services; public, private and voluntary sectors; allopathic and non-allopathic physicians; qualified and unqualified medical practitioners; and multiple health financing systems. There are many areas where this variegated health system has fault lines. Two of the most critical areas are health financing and health workforce (Reddy 2018).

Health Financing

The health system needs to be financed adequately to develop and maintain the required infrastructure, employ an adequate number of skilled health professionals of different categories, pay for procurement of medical products and technologies, ensure efficient administrative and regulatory functions, provide a wide range of health services to the population including health promotion and disease prevention, educate health professionals, fund health research and operate reliable health information systems. Much of these depend on public financing.

The role of public funding becomes especially important when the health system has to ensure wide outreach, easy accessibility, appropriate care for all across the entire life course, and affordability of all health services, to deliver the promise of universal health coverage (UHC). No country has achieved or even approximated UHC without an adequate level of public financing (WHO 2013).

Unfortunately, public financing for health has been stagnant at very low levels for several years in India. It has ranged mostly between 0.9 to 1.2 per cent of the GDP over the past two decades (WHO 2013; World Health Summit 2017). Even if health-relevant expenditures on water and sanitation, and nutrition programmes administered by the Ministry of Women and Child Development are taken into account, public expenditure on health has not gone beyond 1.4 per cent of the GDP in most years. Not only has India's overall per capita health expenditure remained relatively low in comparison to many other countries, but even more disconcertingly, public financing's contribution to that expenditure has been especially low (Table 3.1). Even countries whose overall health expenditure is similar to or lower than India's have a higher fraction of health spending contributed by public financing (World Health Summit 2017).

Table 3.1: Total Health Spending and Governmental Health Spending (2015)

	Total health spending as % of Gross Domestic Product (GDP) 2015	*Government health spending as % of total health spending 2015*
India	3.9	25.6
China	5.3	59.8
Indonesia	3.3	38.2
South Africa	8.2	53.6
Mexico	5.9	52.2
Germany	11.2	84.5
United Kingdom	9.9	80.4
United States	16.8	50.4

Source: Adapted by author from the World Health Statistics Database (2017e) (WHO 2017).

This has resulted in high levels of out-of-pocket spending (OOPS) which impacts adversely on individual and family finances. The poor either deny themselves healthcare because they cannot afford it or risk further impoverishment when they seek much needed care in desperation. Even those who are classified as being above the poverty line are at the risk of being pushed into the poverty abyss by the brute force of high personal expenditure (OOPS). This is particularly true of those just above the poverty line and a substantial section of the middle class. It is not surprising that 7 per cent of Indians experience healthcare-related poverty any year. The estimates of Indians experiencing such poverty have varied between 63 million and 55 million persons over the past decade (Ministry of Health and Family Welfare 2017; Selvaraj, Farooqui and Karan 2018).

Financial vulnerability of individuals seeking healthcare arises from several sources. Direct influences are the costs of hospitalisation, outpatient care and medicines. Outpatient care accounts for 70 per cent of OOPS and medicines account for 70 per cent of the spending on outpatient care (Selvaraj, Farooqui and Karan 2018). Hospitalisation results in sudden demands on family finances and can be catastrophic. Health spending has been called catastrophic when it amounts to an unusually large fraction of a family's monthly income (variably assessed at different thresholds of 10 per cent, 20 per cent or 40 per cent). While such an expenditure can suddenly crush the family into poverty, and therefore alarms economists, chronic financial strain and poverty also result from recurrent or drawn-out outpatient expenditure, draining the family income over a long period. Both forms of health expenditure can lead to indebtedness, sale or mortgaging of even the small farm holdings or homes, and also deprivation of needed education and nutrition for children. Healthcare-related indebtedness has been identified as an important cause of farmer suicides in India.

Apart from these direct expenditures, other causes of financial strain arising from illness care are: lost wages, especially for daily wage workers and others in the informal workforce (with wages often lost also for family caregivers); transport costs (heavy when the healthcare facilities are far away) and not infrequent 'extra payments' that are coercively extracted by healthcare providers or other employees in a healthcare facility. Public financing of assured, easily accessible and appropriate healthcare is essential to overcome these challenges that individuals face when they seek help from the health services. Good governance, too, is essential, to ensure ethical and efficient care, and to prevent physical, emotional and financial maltreatment of care seekers. Ensuring such good management systems, too, needs public financing, since the public healthcare system is the principal source of care for the poor and vulnerable sections of the population.

What should the level of public financing be? It has been suggested by the WHO that ideally, direct payments (OOPS) should not exceed 15–20 per cent of all healthcare expenditure (Evans, David and Etienne 2010). In countries where the role of directly purchased private insurance is low, as in India, the larger fraction of health spending has to come from public financing. If India aims to reduce OOPS even in stages, it must aim to bring it to 50 per cent or lower as the first step. The WHO has estimated that effective implementation of UHC will require 5–6 per cent of the GDP (United Nations Sustainable Development Solutions Network 2015). So, India would need to dedicate 2.5 per cent of the GDP as public financing as an essential first step to be taken by 2020 and then progressively increase it to 3.5 per cent over the next decade. Only then can UHC be achieved by 2030, as mandated by the sustainable development goals (SDG). With the total health expenditure at 5 per cent of the GDP and public financing at a level of 3.5 per cent of the GDP, it would be possible to provide UHC to meet most health needs of the population, while lowering OOPS to 30 per cent. That should not be beyond the scope of a country which is likely to be the world's third largest economy by 2030.

For public financing to rise to that level, both central and state budgets should allocate more for health than they do now. The centre contributes a third of the public funding for health and the states contribute the rest. Therefore, health financing should rise progressively in both the central and state budgets over the next decade. Central budgets have so far not shown an inclination to match the avowed intent to substantially increase the allocation for health. Health allocations show a wide variation in state budgets (Figure 3.1). The National Institution for Transforming India (NITI) Aayog has called for a doubling of percent allocations for health in state budgets between 2017 and 2020 ('8% or above of the total budget') (NITI Aayog 2017). Will the states do so and will the centre show the way? Future budgets will reveal whether the promised rise in public financing will materialise.

Figure 3.1: Per Capita Government Health Expenditure in Indian States (INR) 2018–19

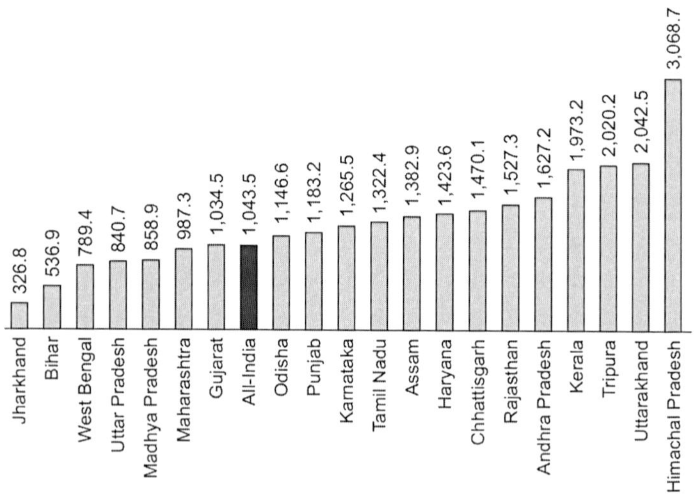

Source: Adapted by author from respective state and central government budget documents (2018–19).

One of the arguments advanced by budget makers, to stall a rise in public financing for health, is that even the money presently allocated for health programmes is not fully utilised. This is a specious argument, since a feeble health system is not capable of utilising the resources fully or optimally. Without considerable investment in infrastructure, health workforce, equipment, drugs and supplies, information technology, management and regulatory systems, many state health systems are not in a position to spend the money allocated through national health programmes. To create stronger health systems, much more core funding is required—well beyond the programme funding. Even to increase the demand for, and utilisation of, health services, the financial barriers to care-seeking must be removed and public confidence must be created that public healthcare facilities are capable of delivering needed services with assured quality. All of this requires greater budgetary allocations for health, both in central and state budgets, to overcome the existing constraints in both supply and demand of health services. To use a Thai simile, trying to push programme funds through a slack health service provision channel is like trying to push a watermelon through a narrow rubber garden hose.

Health Workforce

The WHO includes India in its list of countries which are experiencing a 'health workforce crisis'. The shortages exist across most categories of qualified healthcare providers: doctors (basic and specialist); nurses (graduate and postgraduate, and also auxiliary nurse midwives); and a wide variety of allied health professionals. Health system managers, public health experts and community health workers are also in short supply. Even those who are available are inequitably distributed across states and are mostly concentrated in cities (Figures 3.2 and 3.3).

The production of doctors has been controlled by the Medical Council of India (MCI), which has come under severe criticism from the Supreme Court of India and the Parliamentary Standing Committee on Health. The disbanding of the elected Medical

Figure 3.2: HRH Density across Indian States

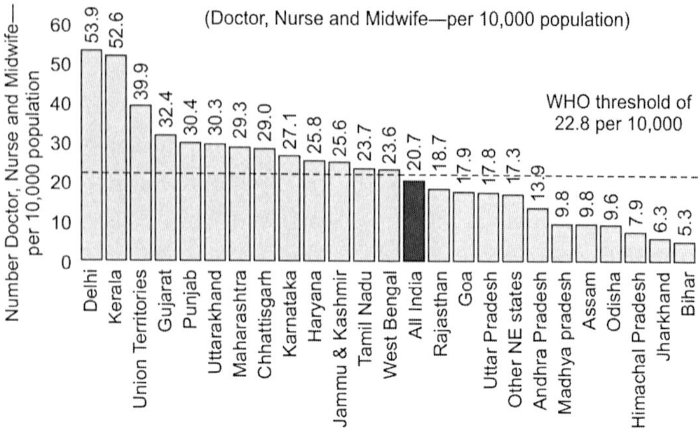

Considering only doctors, nurses and midwives,
HRH density comes out to be 20.7 per 10,000 population

Source: Adapted by author from NSSO 2011–12 data.

Figure 3.3: Rural–Urban Distribution of Health Workforce

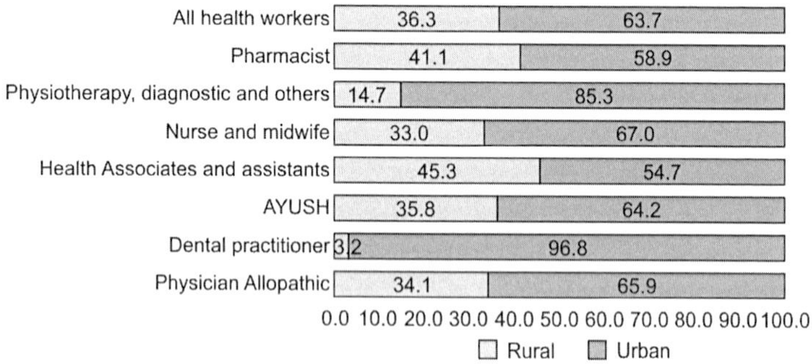

Source: Adapted by author from NSSO 2011–12 data.

Council—twice in the last decade—was forced upon successive governments by the serious public discontent about the functioning of the MCI. The inability of the two ruling dispensations since 2009 to bring about a parliamentary legislation for replacing or supplanting the MCI with a broad-based National Commission on Human Resources in Health (NCHRH) or a narrower National

Medical Commission (NMC) speaks of the lobbying power wielded by those who are resisting reforms.

In her address to the Parliament on 4 June 2009, President Pratibha Patil announced the government's intent to establish the NCHRH (The National Commission for Human Resources for Health Bill 2011) 'as an overarching regulatory body for the health sector to reform the current regulatory framework and enhance supply of skilled personnel'. This was intended to regulate competency-based medical, dental, nursing, pharmacy, public health and allied health professional education, and provide a platform for promoting inter-professional education. Renamed as a Commission rather than a Council, a draft legislation was prepared by the health ministry. This proposal crashed over the rocky terrain of inter-ministerial conflicts (with the Ministry of Human Resources Development wanting to regulate all of higher education), revision by successive health ministry committees, and a critical review by the Parliamentary Standing Committee on Health. An attempt to instead enact amendments to the MCI Act failed when forces aligned to the entrenched leadership of the MCI forced a retreat.

Caustic observations of the Supreme Court of India on the flaws and failings of the MCI, and the medical profession's dismay at the Council's growing disrepute, triggered a fresh initiative by the present government to reform medical education through a bill for replacing the MCI with the NMC. The bill's intent was laudable as it sought to free medical education from regressive regulatory cobwebs and strengthen both healthcare and health research. However, protests by the Indian Medical Association (IMA) and concerns expressed by even supporters of the reform over the lacunae in some provisions led to the bill being referred to the Parliamentary Standing Committee on Health for its review. Though that Committee provided some recommendations to address these concerns, the redrafted bill has not been presented to the Parliament. The MCI was again disbanded in September 2018 and an empowered committee was constituted by the government to regulate medical education. The approach of successive governments has been akin to a doctor prescribing an anti-pyretic when the fever peaks but not to attempt a remedy that can cure the main ailment. The yo-yo cycle of dissolution and restoration of a discredited MCI continues in cycles of fluctuating potential response to the lobbying power of MCI establishment and the countervailing force of public and judicial criticism. Real reform still awaits!

The main cause of erosion of values in medical education is the subversion of the social role of medical education by corruption. This has manifested in many forms—from the licensing and re-licensing of medical colleges which are ill-equipped to impart quality education to the outrageously exorbitant capitation fees collected for the admission of students in private medical colleges.

Much of this drift has occurred after private, for-profit medical colleges started proliferating over the last four decades. Of the 468 medical colleges functioning, 259 are privately owned and managed. Of these, 105 have opened since 2010 (Potnuru 2017). Medical education became a business linked to large profits and disengaged from its social mission. Powerful political and business interests converged to create new colleges that can charge huge sums from aspirant students. Regulators often turned a blind eye to distortions and deficiencies in several of these institutions, either passively caving in under political pressure or actively colluding due to pecuniary temptations.

The role of money as the vehicle of corruption, used for hijacking medical education through flawed licensing, is difficult to prove, though generally considered a prevalent reality. However, falsification of faculty strength and patient admission numbers, to befool complacent or complicit inspectors who visit medical colleges, has been widely reported upon. False faculty rosters, with non-existent persons listed to meet the regulatory requirements, are familiar stories. Frequently, the same individuals are listed as full-time faculty in several institutions at the same time. Part-time faculty are shown as full-time employees, even though the salary slips indicate only a limited engagement. Reports abound of planted 'patients' who are hired for the day to fill vacant beds to create the facade of a hospital functioning to full capacity. Private medical college managers have been known to hire agents who supply such pseudo-patients at inspection time. Inspectors may be conned or even cynically connive to clear such colleges despite their inability to truly qualify. Ghost faculty and guest artist 'patients' thus carry the day, and colleges continue to enrol students despite the lack of adequate faculty and facilities for training.

In March 2016, the Parliamentary Standing Committee on Health and Family Welfare submitted its report evaluating the performance of the MCI and recommending reforms in the regulation of medical education. The concluding chapter (Ministry of Health and Family Welfare 2016) opens thus: 'The Committee observes that the Medical Council of India as the regulator of India in the country has repeatedly failed on all its mandates over the years'. Among the several shortcomings listed, is 'Failure to create a transparent system of medical college inspections and grant of recognition or de-recognition', and 'Failure to put in place a robust quality assurance mechanism' (ibid.).

Admission of students to private, for-profit medical colleges comes with a hefty price tag. Termed as the capitation fee, it is the purchase price of medical education when marks in the qualifying examination do not earn students admission into a government-run or not-for-profit private medical college. This is considered legitimate, though courts have insisted on a merit-based admission within this high-paying category. Some private medical colleges also have a management quota which carries a premium price. Apart from listed capitation fees, high as it is, there is also the frequent demand for under-the-table payment, which is not reported as income. Capitation fees—with both revealed and hidden components—has become the exorbitantly expensive entry ticket for students seeking admission to both undergraduate and postgraduate degree programmes in the for-profit private medical colleges. Students who pay vast sums of money—with a rumoured fee of Rs 3–4 crores for admittance to sought-after postgraduate courses like radiology—are likely to seek quick recovery of their investment through inappropriate medical practice. In a lucrative branch like radiology, it is indeed an ultrasound investment, when you scan it! Unfortunately, this conveyor belt of corruption leads from college to clinic, with a cynical discard of morals in education and ethics in practice, along the way.

Even government medical colleges are not fully free of unethical behaviour. Most of the government-run medical colleges in the country permit private practice by the clinical faculty. When preoccupation with that practice becomes overwhelming, commitment to clinical teaching suffers. This is not financial corruption, but dereliction of teaching duties is moral corruption. Such behaviours also create wrong role models for students.

The unmasking of a decade-old admission scam in Madhya Pradesh in 2009 revealed the ugly face of rampant and systematically organised corruption in examinations conducted for selection to pre-medical and postgraduate medical courses. The Madhya Pradesh Professional Examination Board (MPPEB) was better known by its Hindi acronym, '*Vyapam*'. Investigations since 2013 revealed the involvement of several politicians, bureaucrats, MPPEB officials, racketeers, agents, candidates and parents, and led to the arrest of more than 2,000 persons by 2015. Among the courses determined to have been rigged were pre-medical tests (2008–13) and the postgraduate selection test of 2012. Methods employed ranged from impersonation of candidates to falsification of marks. Over 40 of the accused persons or witnesses have died since under mysterious circumstances, with the Special Investigating Team of the police declaring 23 of these deaths to be unnatural (Rout 2015).

The ills that have plagued medical education have also afflicted dental and nursing education, with suspect regulatory bodies, widely varying standards of education across the colleges, and the overwhelming desire of private investors to reap vast profits from commercial models of professional education, unmindful of the quality of training imparted. Unfortunately, regulatory reform has not touched these areas of health professional education. The training of allied health professionals (previously referred to as paramedical streams) is another area of policy inertia or vacillation. Many of the categories of allied health professionals have no accrediting body or standardised courses. An attempt to set up an overarching council for a range of allied health professional training programmes has gone into hibernation within the government. An earlier proposal to set up the National Institute of Paramedical Sciences and eight Regional Institutes of Paramedical Sciences has also dropped off the radar, with the proposal for the regional institutes reportedly given up and the national institute still a work in slow progress.

Service Provision: Public and Private

A mixed health system has evolved in India, by default and not by design. The role of the public sector, dominant in the first 35 years after Independence, declined in importance over time due to low levels of funding and poor management. The private sector, on the other hand, has grown rapidly during the last 35 years, with corporate chains and large urban hospitals springing up with the help of private financing and government concessions. While in the initial years of independent India, the public sector provided most of the care, the private sector now provides 80 per cent of the outpatient care and 60 per cent of the inpatient care (Loh, Ugarte-Gil and Darko 2013). The private sector is a mixed bag of world-class tertiary care centres, single speciality hospitals, general nursing homes, family-run clinics and individual practitioners (qualified and unqualified). The public sector has a three-tier primary healthcare system (with sub, primary and community health centres), district hospitals and medical college hospitals. Recently, many clones of the prestigious All-India Institute of Medical Sciences, New Delhi, have been coming up in different states. Despite bearing the same name, many of these new institutes are struggling to find faculty and grow to full potential.

Weaknesses in the public sector are noted across the entire chain of facilities, from sub-centres to medical college hospitals. This has been principally due to inadequate investment in infrastructure, human resources and equipment, compounded by poor management. In most states, doctors employed in public hospitals are allowed to do private practice, with large portions of their time and attention diverted to that pursuit. Poor pay scales in the public sector do little to encourage commitment and retention. Public sector health services in Tamil Nadu, the All-India Railway Medical Services and Armed Forces Medical Services are shining examples. However, in most states, the public sector presents a picture of malaise traceable to poor public policy, inadequate monitoring and low accountability. Devoted doctors are still found in the public sector, but the system has failed them.

The private sector has flourished due to the void created by the dwindling capacity and competence of the public sector and aided by a weak regulatory environment. The inability of many states to even adopt and implement the Clinical Establishments Act is evidence of their yielding to the power and influence of the private sector. The large corporate hospitals, too, have come under fire in the media because of the high cost of care and instances of shocking insensitivity to human suffering due to crass commercial considerations. There are several sections of the private sector that do practise ethical medicine, performing commendable humanitarian service, and many who combine the best of science and skills to deliver healthcare at the summit of global standards. However, the lack of a regulatory system creates a permissive atmosphere which allows the delinquents to overshadow the dedicated.

There is a need to optimally utilise the resources of both the public sector and the private sector (with its for-profit and not-for-profit segments) to deliver needed health services across this vast land. The models of public–private partnership (PPP) deployed so far have not worked well, for several reasons. Poorly designed contracts, vaguely defined deliverables and inadequately enforced accountability have frequently led to failures in service delivery, especially to the poor. The dependence on the private sector for service delivery in government-funded health insurance schemes in the past 15 years has yielded valuable lessons on how unregulated partnerships can lead to unintended consequences of induced demand and unnecessary procedures. As Ayushman Bharat (National Portal of India n.d.) launches an even more ambitious programme of cost coverage of hospitalisation, with private hospital empanelment, it is essential to design partnership frameworks and regulatory systems which can keep public interest uppermost, maximise coverage and efficiencies while minimising distortions in cost and quality of care. The civil society often defines PPP as 'partnership for private profit'. It is necessary that the government earnestly redefines it as 'partnership for public purpose' in the context of UHC, clearly delineating the deliverables and the accountability measures (Reddy 2017). The best guarantee for ensuring that a private sector partner imbibes the public purpose and plays by the rules is to strengthen the public sector so that it can set benchmarks in cost optimisation and quality of service delivery, hence the need for greater public financing for health.

References

2011. Clauses AOF, Ii C, Iii C. *The National Commission for Human Resources for Health Bill.*

de Savigny, D., and T. Adam. 2009. 'Systems Thinking for Health Systems Strengthening'. Geneva. Available at https://apps.who.int/iris/bitstream/handle/10665/44204/9789241563895_eng.pdf;jsessionid=A53089D8DB64F5AC3DC217F3D809938F?sequence=1 (accessed 22 February 2019).

Evans, David B., and C. Etienne. 2010. 'The World Health Report: Health Systems Financing'. World Health Organization, 1–128.

Loh, L. C., C. Ugarte-Gil, and K. Darko. 2013. 'Private Sector Contributions and their Effect on Physician Emigration in the Developing World'. *Bull World Health Organ* 91 (3): 227–33.

Ministry of Health and Family Welfare. 2016. 'Ninety-Second Department-related Parliamentary Standing Committee on the Functioning of Medical Council of India'.

Ministry of Health and Family Welfare. 2017. 'National Health Policy 2017'. New Delhi. Available at http://cdsco.nic.in/writereaddata/National-Health-Policy.pdf (accessed 16 November 2018).

National Portal of India. n.d. 'Ayushman Bharat—National Health Protection Mission'. Available at https://www.india.gov.in/spotlight/ayushman-bharat-national-health-protection-mission (accessed 13 November 2018).

NITI Aayog. 2017. 'India: Three Year Action Agenda 2017–2018 to 2019–2020'. Available at http://niti.gov.in/writereaddata/files/coop/IndiaActionPlan.pdf (accessed 11 November 2018).

Potnuru, B. 2017. 'Aggregate Availability of Doctors in India: 2014–2030'. *Indian J Public Health* 61 (3): 182–87.

Reddy, K. S. 2017. 'How to Define Public Purpose for a PPP to Move Beyond Marriage of Convenience; Here is what is Critically Crucial'. *Financial Express*, 13 July. Available at http://www.financialexpress.com/opinion/how-to-define-public-purpose-for-a-ppp-to-move-beyond-marriage-of-convenience-here-is-what-is-critically-crucial/761151/ (accessed 16 November 2018).

_____. 2018. 'Health Care Reforms in India'. *Journal of the American Medical Association* 319 (24): 2477–78.

Rout, S. 2015. 'All You Need to Know about the Vyapam Scam that is Killing People'. *Business Standard*. Available at http://www.business-standard.com/article/politics/all-you-need-to-know-about-the-vyapam-scam-that-is-killing-people-115070600446_1.html (accessed 18 November 2018).

Selvaraj, S., H. H. Farooqui, and A. Karan. 2018. 'Quantifying the Financial Burden of Households' Out-of-Pocket Payments on Medicines in India: A Repeated Cross-sectional Analysis of National Sample Survey Data, 1994–2014'. *BMJ Open* 8 (5): e018020.

United Nations Sustainable Development Solutions Network. 2015. 'Financing Universal Health Coverage in the Post-2015 Agenda'. *Themat Gr Heal All* 24: 1–11.

World Health Organization. 2000. 'The World Health Report 2000: Health Systems: Improving Performance'. Geneva. Available at http://www.who.int/whr/2000/en/whr00_en.pdf (accessed 16 November 2018).

World Health Organization. 2013. 'Arguing for Universal Health Coverage'. Geneva. Available at https://apps.who.int/iris/bitstream/handle/10665/204355/9789241506342_eng.pdf?sequence=1&isAllowed=y (accessed 11 November 2018).

_____. 2017. 'World Health Statistics'. Available at https://www.who.int/gho/publications/world_health_statistics/2017/en/ (accessed 18 November 2018).

World Health Summit. 2017. Available at https://www.worldhealthsummit.org/about/history/2017.html (accessed 11 November 2018).

four

Access to Medicines

> Many governments have not used the flexibilities available under the TRIPS agreement for various reasons ranging from capacity constraints to undue political and economic pressure from states and corporations, both express and implied. Political and economic pressures placed on governments to forgo the use of TRIPS flexibilities violates the integrity and legitimacy of the system of legal rights and duties created by the TRIPS Agreement, as reaffirmed by the Doha Declaration.
>
> UN High Level Panel

'Of the 55 million Indians who became poor due to healthcare expenditure in 2011–2012, 38 million were impoverished because of spending on medicines' (Selvaraj, Farooqui and Karan 2018). This revelation may come as a shock to all who see India as a producer of inexpensive drugs. Indeed, India has become reputed as the 'global pharmacy', with both branded and unbranded generics finding large export markets. Why, then, the poverty created by medicines in India?

While the low purchasing capacity of a large segment of the Indian population may be a factor contributing to this paradox, the main reason is that many drugs in India are priced higher than they should be. While a reasonable level of profit is acceptable as a market mechanism, high mark-ups over the manufacturing cost make the drugs costlier than they need to be and impose undue burden on the consumer.

Pharmaceutical products have been a major ally of modern medicine and have provided the ability to cure disease, save and prolong lives, provide relief and even prevent some diseases. Their availability and affordability are, therefore, essential elements of a health system and a key consideration for health policy. However, this is an area where public interest and corporate profit-maximising behaviours have clashed frequently. The government has a duty to ensure that needed medicines are easily available and that cost does not become a barrier to their use, even while providing the pharmaceutical industry with the opportunities and incentives to produce and market needed drugs in rational formulations. The government must also be an effective regulator of quality, price and promotional methods.

Prices and Patents

The multinational manufacturers have traditionally charged high prices, citing the high costs of development research, testing and trials as the reasons for extracting high retail prices. These arguments have been countered by exposures of how much of the initial drug development process has been driven by publicly funded academic research and how high post-development prices reflect the costs of unduly expensive trials followed by extravagant advertising and promotion (Angell 2005; Goldacre 2012). The high profit margins which are tagged to patented products are fiercely protected by battles to stretch the patents as they are set to expire.

Multinational pharmaceutical companies faced their first major challenge in India when the country adopted 'process patenting' instead of 'product patenting' in the regulatory system. This landmark move, enacted by the Indian Parliament in 1970, gave fillip to the Indian generic industry, which then grew by leaps and bounds (Government of India 1970). This enabled the many previously patent-protected drugs to be produced in a generic form, through an altered process of manufacture, and allowed the drugs to be sold at a far lower price than the patented brands. The multinationals fought this, but the Indian law protected and promoted the Indian industry. Some multinationals quit the Indian market, but others lowered their prices to stay and sell in the country. Some even adopted the practice of buying from the generic manufacturers, packaging under their own brand names, and marketing at a price considerably higher than the generic price, but lower than their previous branded price. So much for brand value!

India's population size offers a huge market for foreign drug manufacturers and the country's economic growth projects a large middle class which can buy drugs (PWC 2010). So, even firms that quit in pique over the process patenting policy have returned to explore and access the profits that the Indian market now has to offer. New methods adopted by some multinational drug companies include tiered pricing set at lower rates for the Indian market, franchising of production to domestic generic manufacturers for India-restricted manufacture and marketing at lower than international prices. For example, the anti-hepatitis drug sofosbuvir has been franchised to several domestic drug manufacturers, for manufacture and sale at a small fraction of the international price (*The Times of India* 2017). The latest is an offer to the Government of India, by the US-India Business Council, which promotes the interests of multinational drug manufacturers, to offer their products for use in the Ayushman Bharat programme at a special discounted price (Dey 2018). This will enable them to get access to a large publicly financed programme, with an assured market, while protecting the open market sale of their products from price control.

The Indian manufacturers would like to protect their right to produce generics, fighting the multinational manufacturers who attempt to curtail that right through legal battles. However, the Indian manufacturers of branded generics resent and resist price control on their products, many of which have high mark-ups. Thus, while they have greatly benefited from the 'process patenting' regime introduced in the 1970s, they are now not fully ready to pass the benefit to the Indian consumers of their products.

Price control is a fiercely contested policy instrument, both in the method of price fixation and in the purported impact on availability of the drugs whose price is controlled. The Indian government weighed its options between 'cost plus' and 'market average' methods, but settled for the latter, much to the relief of the drug manufacturers and dismay of the public health community (Narula 2015). The 'cost plus' method estimates the actual cost of manufacture and adds a permissible profit margin to arrive at a reasonable fixed price for sale. The mechanism of cost-plus-based pricing was followed for fixing ceiling prices of formulations by taking into account the raw material cost, conversion cost, packaging material cost and packing charges. A maximum allowable post-manufacturing expenses was allowed over and above these costs, to the extent of 100 per cent (Selvaraj, Farooqui and Mehta 2019). The central idea of 'market-based pricing' was to compute the ceiling price of a specific formulation under the National List of Essential Medicines (NLEM) by taking a simple average of the prices to retailers of all brands, with a market share equal to or greater than 1 per cent of the overall market for the said formulation and adding a retailer's margin of 16 per cent to obtain the maximum retail price (ibid.). High-selling 'reputed' brands which carry high sale price prior to this calculation can skew the derived average. This leads to prices higher than would be arrived at by the 'cost plus' method. It also permits the manufacturers who were charging low prices (below this average price) to move their products to the higher price cap, as the average price is now advantageous to them. India moved from cost plus pricing to market-based pricing of NLEM products in 2013.

The pharmaceutical industry argues against price control by asserting that the manufacturers lose interest in producing price-controlled drugs and people would be the losers as a result. This suggests that profit trumps the public purpose for these manufacturers, who are not satisfied with the margin of profit offered by the 'cost plus' method of price fixation. This can become a pressure tactic, where there is little or no public sector capacity to manufacture essential drugs and the health system is mostly or wholly dependent on the willingness of the private sector for the production and supply of these drugs. Unfortunately, much of the public sector capacity in the manufacture of drugs and vaccines has disappeared or dwindled in the last four decades. This leaves the health policy very vulnerable to industry tactics, which resist and reject substantial price controls, since no responsible government can allow the needed drugs to disappear from the market.

While the foreign and Indian drug manufacturers are cordially united in resisting price control, they spiritedly contest each other in the arena of patent rights. The foreign holders of the patent try various methods to prolong the patent beyond its expiry date and claim 'data exclusivity' to deny the generic manufacturer access to the clinical trial data that proved the drug's efficacy and safety (Diependaele, Cockbain and Sterckx 2017). When the Indian manufacturers of generic drugs contest these moves, they gain the support of civil society organisations, which advocate patient rights. The nature of alliances changes, based on whether the Indian drug industry is combating governmental regulations or barriers placed by international competitors.

It is a generally agreed principle that data related to proof of efficacy of a drug, based on clinical trials, need not be provided afresh when approval is sought for registration of a generic drug after the patent on the original product has expired. In such cases, the regulatory agency relies on the original evidence of efficacy and safety, as also on the evidence of bioequivalence between the generic and original forms. By demanding data exclusivity, large manufacturers deny access to the original evidence of efficacy that can support the claim of the generic and thereby kill competition that can lower drug prices. This is an attempt to effectively extend the patent on the branded drug, even after the patent has legally expired. The Declaration of Helsinki (Mihajlovic-Madzarevic 2010), a charter of reference on bio-ethics, states that conducting duplicative clinical trials on human subjects is unethical when the question of efficacy has already been settled. Further, denial of original trial data can block a decision by any government to issue a compulsory licence to a generic manufacturer in response to a public health imperative, as permitted by the World Trade Organization (WTO).

'Ever greening' is a favoured technique of patent prolongation, wherein new patents are sought, on associated delivery system or new pharmaceutical mixtures, of a product whose patent is soon to expire (Shukla 2011). This is not permissible by law, but the patent holder still claims this modification to be a new product. This is a method by which the manufacturer seeks to gain patent extension of the original product by attaching the name to modified product which has a different formulation (such as a dose change to a higher strength or change from a pill to a powder) or using the drug in combination with another drug and demanding further patent protection.

Drug prices are also linked to the patent rights protected by the WTO. The Agreement on Trade Related Intellectual Property

Rights (TRIPS Agreement) (WTO, TRIPS 1994), originally developed to harmonise patent regimes across the world, has been used to contest generic production of patented products. TRIPS gave wide latitude to developed countries housing multinational drug manufacturers to decide on conditions under which patents could be granted. This enabled them to support practices such as ever greening and block generic manufacturers in developing countries. The resultant access barriers to essential and life-saving drugs, which compromised the health of developing country populations, led to protests against this imposed inequity. The Doha Declaration of 2001 (WHO 2015) emerged from this debate, with provisions for 'compulsory licensing' and 'parallel importation', which gave precedence to public health over commercial rights. Countries such as India, Brazil and Thailand have benefited from this.

The Doha Declaration stresses that TRIPS 'can and should be interpreted and implemented' to support the 'right to protect public health [and] promote access to medicines for all', including the sovereign determination of the grounds under which a compulsory licence may be issued (WHO 2015). Governments must review the situation of access to health technologies in their countries in light of human rights principles and states' obligations to fulfil them.

Compulsory licensing for the manufacture of medicinal products is when a government allows a drug manufacturer (located within its jurisdiction) to produce a patented product or process without the consent of the patent owner or plans to use the patent itself. The patent owner is paid a fee, but has no right to deny or block the grant of the production right by the government. This right has been exercised by developing countries in case of public health emergencies and for the production of life-saving medicines. A government may use this right sparingly, but must have the domestic capacity to produce drugs under that right. The Indian private drug manufacturers can use that license when provided by the government. However, the growing trend of foreign drug companies acquiring Indian firms may narrow that channel. Other Indian firms may wish to avoid the threat of litigation or coercive tactics of foreign governments aligned to multinationals. What would happen if no private drug company in India is ready, for whatever reasons, to undertake manufacture under a compulsory license? The government must ensure that enough public sector capacity is available to undertake such manufacture—all the more the need for greater governmental investment in reviving the public sector capacity for the manufacture of medicines and vaccines.

However, new trade agreements have been initiated by developed countries to bypass the WTO and restrict the flexibilities provided by the Doha Declaration. A number of Free Trade Agreements (FTAs) have been mooted by developed countries to introduce restrictions beyond those envisaged in the WTO agreements and have separate dispute settlement mechanisms that go beyond the inter-governmental process. The provisions include 'data exclusivity', curbs on 'compulsory licensing' and involvement of the pharmaceutical industry in dispute settlement. The 'Investor State Dispute Settlement' (ISDS) gives an opportunity to a corporate investor in a product to engage a government in litigation over patent and trade issues. This has already been misused by the tobacco industry in attempts to block tobacco control measures. The ISDS enables industries to drag governments to court by launching vexatious litigation on matters related to generic drug production and price control. Some FTA provisions will also allow high-income countries to seize drugs from generic drug manufacturing countries during transit to other countries (on suspicion of intellectual property being violated). For example, seizure of generic drugs exported by India to another developing country, while in transit through a developed country, can also become an imminent threat under the FTA if such provisions are accepted.

The main argument that is advanced to defend such measures, which restrict treatment access to poor patients across the world, is that protection of intellectual property is the sacred duty of governments. The case is made that large pharmaceutical companies invest a huge amount of money in the research and development of new drugs, and patent protection offers them the only opportunity to recover those costs. However, it has been well-documented that much of the initial foundational research in drug development comes from publicly funded work at universities and research institutes and that pharmaceutical companies access rights to that work from the public domain (or through permissive pathways such as the Bayh-Dole Act of United States) (Angell 2005; ORI n.d.). The costs of further drug development and testing, incurred by the pharmaceutical firms, do not justify the super-profits earned on many of the patented drugs.

India needs to protect its vital interests in any trade agreement, just as other nations strive to. Our interest lies in protecting the lives and safeguarding the health of Indians without permitting unreasonable restrictions on our ability to produce, use, and even export, generic versions of drugs, the patents of which have lapsed (or where compulsory licensing has been invoked to protect public health). India needs to tread carefully while negotiating an FTA with any other country, so that the health of the Indian people is not compromised through provisions that shackle our generic drug industry.

Another measure that must accompany the production and promotion of generic drugs is that they must be prescribed by doctors, in preference over higher priced branded products. The

Government of India and the MCI announced in 2017 that doctors would be mandated to write prescriptions using only the generic names of the drugs (Medical Council of India n.d.). Prescription of drugs by their generic name will curtail the physician's habit of prescribing a costly brand when a cheaper yet effective alternative is available. The unwary patient must not, however, be beguiled by a canny pharmacist who misuses the generic prescription to sell the brand which provides the highest profit margin, ignoring the cheaper alternatives. For this, public and patient education (generic drug literacy) must be promoted so that patients or their family members can easily refer to the manufacturer and price listings of the alternatives available under each generic name. Such a catalogue, periodically updated, must be displayed in a touch-screen format (in English, Hindi and a regional language) in each pharmacy. Any purchaser should be able to choose from this menu and estimate the cost before purchasing. Computerised sales records must be randomly surveyed periodically to ensure that pharmacists are not preferentially favouring drugs in the higher price range. Combination drugs, which mingle two or more generic medicines in a single tablet or capsule, must be closely scrutinised for rationale, pharmacokinetics and efficacy. Generic prescriptions will reduce the scope for their misuse.

This also imposes a responsibility on the part of the government to ensure that only quality-assured generics are sold. Substandard drugs need to be continually weeded out. The number and quality of drug testing and certification laboratories must increase. Domestic production of generics must be boosted, as indeed of the basic chemicals that are needed for pharmaceutical production. Dependency on other countries for import of those chemicals will mean that our domestic generic industry can be held hostage by the exporting country, for political or commercial reasons, and a sudden blockade of that supply chain can catastrophically cut down our pharmaceutical production.

Procurement and Supply Chain

A pooled procurement mechanism is best used for reducing drug prices when bulk purchase of drugs is needed for public sector use. Quality-assured generics can thereby be obtained at low prices directly from the manufacturer, eliminating multiple layers of mark-up that lie on the road to retail. Tamil Nadu and Rajasthan have shown how this works well and why states should adopt this practice (Mukherjee 2014). Private sector hospitals, too, can be encouraged to buy from autonomous central or state procurement agencies, which follow this method, and pass on the benefit to their patients. As Ayushman Bharat is implemented, the empanelled hospitals (both public and private sector) may be mandated to purchase only through such agencies which can efficiently negotiate prices through the pooled public procurement process.

Procurement will be ineffective in benefiting the patients if supply chain management is poor. Quite often, stock-outs occur at the point of drug dispensing, for example primary or community health centres. Since the proposed Health and Wellness Centres under Ayushman Bharat (Government of India 2018) will also become drug-dispensing facilities for several essential drugs, it is all the more necessary to have an efficient supply chain. Tamil Nadu has shown how this can be effectively done through district warehouses and information technology-enabled monitoring of drug dispensing and stock positions at each healthcare facility. Once well established, these systems can also be used for post-marketing surveillance of the adverse effects of drugs.

The Jan Aushadi chain of generic drug stores (BPPI, Government of India 2017), promoted by the government, can also be effective in ensuring the availability of generic drugs at affordable prices in many parts of the country. This will enable even a person purchasing drugs prescribed by private doctors to avoid high out-of-pocket expenditure. When combined with free distribution of drugs at public healthcare facilities, this can greatly reduce the presently high financial burden of medicines on individuals and families.

Engagement in Shaping Global Agreements

There is also a need to engage with global trade regulations, both to protect our right to produce essential drugs and our ability to export generics. A report of the United Nations High Level Panel on Innovation and Access to Health Technologies (2016) called upon countries to safeguard and fully utilise the rights conferred by the TRIPS flexibilities, as confirmed by the Doha Declaration of the WTO (United Nations 2016). It asks WTO members to resist and report any political or economic pressure exerted to subvert these rights. It cautions against the threat posed to the rights by FTAs, which introduce provisions to steal the right to resort to compulsory licensing for public health purposes or open the door to industry interference through insertion of ISDS mechanisms.

Further, the UN report also urges member states of the WTO to adopt a permanent revision of paragraph 6 of the TRIPS agreement (WTO, TRIPS 1994) 'to enable swift and expeditious export of pharmaceutical products produced under compulsory licence'. Will India, as the 'pharmacy of the world', take up the global leadership role in making this happen? By doing so, India will improve access and affordability of medicines across the whole world.

References

Angell, M. 2005. *The Truth About the Drug Companies: How They Deceive Us and What to Do About It*. New York: Random House Trade Paperback.

Bureau of Pharma PSUs of India (BPPI), Government of India. 2017. Available at http://janaushadhi.gov.in/index.aspx (accessed 14 January 2019).

Dey, S. 2018. 'Big Pharma Companies Propose Launch of Low Priced "Second Brands" for Ayushman Bharat Health Insurance Scheme'. *The Times of India*, 16 October. Available at https://timesofindia.indiatimes.com/india/big-pharma-proposes-launch-of-low-priced-second-brands-for-ayushman-bharat-health-insurance-scheme/articleshow/66229879.cms (accessed 7 December 2018).

Diependaele, L., J. Cockbain, and S. Sterckx. 2017. 'Raising the Barriers to Access to Medicines in the Developing World—The Relentless Push for Data Exclusivity'. *Dev World Bioeth* 17 (1): 11–21.

Goldacre, B. 2012. *Bad Pharma: How Drug Companies Mislead Doctors and Harm Patients*. London: Fourth Estate.

Government of India. 1970. *The Patents Act, 1970*. Available at https://www.wipo.int/edocs/lexdocs/laws/en/in/in065en.pdf (accessed 8 January 2019).

———. 2018. 'Ayushman Bharat—National Health Protection Mission'. National Portal of India. Available at https://www.india.gov.in/spotlight/ayushman-bharat-national-health-protection-mission (accessed 14 January 2019).

Life Sciences. 2010. 'Global Pharma Looks to India: Prospects for Growth'. PWC. Available at https://www.pwc.com/gx/en/pharma-life-sciences/pdf/global-pharma-looks-to-india-final.pdf (accessed 12 January 2019).

Medical Council of India. n.d. '1.5—Use of Generic names of Drugs'. Available at http://www.ipgmer.gov.in/PharmacovigilanceCommittee/MCI_CircularUseofGenericNames20170421.pdf (accessed 12 Janury 2019).

Mihajlovic-Madzarevic, V. 2010. 'Appendix C: World Medical Association Declaration of Helsinki Ethical Principles for Medical Research Involving Human Subjects', in *Clinical Trials Audit Preparation*,

225–29. Available at https://www.who.int/bulletin/archives/79(4)373.pdf (accessed 21 January 2019).

Mukherjee, R. 2014. 'Unbranded Generics Way to Cheaper Cure'. *The Times of India*, 18 January. Available at https://timesofindia.indiatimes.com/business/india-business/Unbranded-generics-way-to-cheaper-cure/articleshow/28970795.cms (accessed 14 January 2019).

Narula, S. 2015. 'Current Drug Pricing Status in India'. *Pharmacoeconomics* 1 (1): e101.

n.d. 'Bayh-Dole Act' (Public Law: 96–517). ORI—The Office of Research Integrity. Available at https://ori.hhs.gov/content/Chapter-5-Conflicts-of-Interest-bayh-dole-act-public-law-96-517 (accessed 12 January 2019).

Selvaraj, S., H. H. Farooqui, and A. Karan. 2018. 'Quantifying the Financial Burden of Households' Out-of-pocket Payments on Medicines in India: A Repeated Cross-sectional Analysis of National Sample Survey data, 1994–2014'. *BMJ Open* 8 (5): e018020.

Selvaraj, S., H. Farooqui, and A. Mehta. 2019. 'Does Price Regulation Affect Atorvastatin Sales in India? An Impact Assessment through Interrupted Time Series Analysis'. *BMJ Open* 9 (1): e024200.

Shukla, U. 2011. 'Ever Greening Patents'. *Sci Report* 3 (AUGUST): 31–34.

The Times of India. 2017. 'Natco Launches Sofosbuvir Generic', 9 May. Available at https://timesofindia.indiatimes.com/business/india-business/natco-launches-sofosbuvir-generic/articleshow/58583198.cms (accessed 7 January 2019).

United Nations. 2016. 'The United Nations Secretary-General's High-Level Panel on Access to Medicines Report Promoting Innovation and Access to Health Technologies'. New York.

WHO. 2015. The Doha Declaration on the TRIPS Agreement and Public Health. World Health Organization.

WTO, TRIPS. 1994. Annex 1C Agreement on Trade-Related Aspects of Intellectual Property Rights Part I General Provisions and Basic Principles Part II Standards Concerning the Availability, Scope and Use of Intellectual Property Rights. TRIPS Agreem. 319–51.

five

First Steps to Universal Health Coverage

Firm, but not Full or Fast

> Primary care provides a place to which people can bring a wide range of health problems–it is not acceptable that in low income countries primary care would only deal with a few 'priority diseases'.
>
> World Health Report 2008 (WHO 2008)

The poor state of India's health became all too evident when the country began the steep climb to reach the Millennium Development Goals (MDGs) adopted at the United Nations in 2000. The high rates of maternal and child mortality, and the huge burdens of malaria, tuberculosis and HIV-AIDS placed India in the list of countries whose health systems had failed to deliver the benefits of development to the vulnerable sections of the population. Lack of easy access to quality-assured health services was a constant challenge that people had to face in many parts of India. The high out-of-pocket expenditure, which made healthcare unaffordable to many, also highlighted the failure of public policy to recognise its governance responsibility to the people, of protecting their right to health. In 2004, only 21 per cent of the health expenditure in the country came from public financing. About 7 per cent of the population were pushed into poverty due to unaffordable healthcare expenditure (NSSO 2006).

The first major attempt to remedy this sorry state of the health services came through two different initiatives. The National Rural Health Mission (NRHM) attempted to strengthen the ability of the health system to address the needs of maternal and child health, and also infectious disease control, in the larger rural segment of the population. A set of government-financed health insurance schemes were also launched by some states and the central government to provide better access and some financial relief to the economically disadvantaged and vulnerable sections of the population. The chief of these was the Rashtriya Swasthya Bima Yojana (RSBY) or the National Health Insurance Scheme.

The National Rural Health Mission

The NRHM was launched on 12 April 2005.

Objectives of the NRHM (Ministry of Health and Family Welfare 2005)

The mission started with several clearly stated objectives:

- reduction in child and maternal mortality;
- universal access to public services for food and nutrition, sanitation and hygiene, and universal access to public healthcare services with emphasis on services addressing women and children's health and universal immunisation;
- prevention and control of communicable and non-communicable diseases, including locally endemic diseases;
- access to integrated comprehensive primary healthcare;
- population stabilisation, gender and demographic balance;
- revitalisation of local health traditions and mainstream AYUSH (Ayurveda, Yoga, Unani, Siddha and Homeopathy);
- promotion of healthy lifestyles.

Expected Outcomes from the Mission

The outcomes anticipated were:

- IMR reduced to 30/1,000 live births by 2012;
- Maternal Mortality reduced to 100/1,00,000 live births by 2012;
- Total Fertility Rate reduced to 2.1 by 2012;
- Malaria Mortality Reduction Rate: 50 per cent up to 2010, additional 10 per cent by 2012;
- Kala Azar Mortality Reduction Rate: 100 per cent by 2010 and sustaining elimination until 2012;
- Filaria/Microfilaria Reduction Rate: 70 per cent by 2010, 80 per cent by 2012 and elimination by 2015;
- Dengue Mortality Reduction Rate: 50 per cent by 2010 and sustaining at that level until 2012;
- Cataract operations: rising to 46 lakhs until 2012;
- Leprosy Prevalence Rate: reduce from 1.8 per 10,000 in 2005 to less than 1 per 10,000 thereafter;
- Tuberculosis DOTS series: maintain 85 per cent cure rate through entire mission period and also sustain planned case detection rate;
- upgrading all Community Health Centres to Indian public health standards;
- increased utilisation of first referral units, from bed occupancy by referred cases, from less than 20 per cent to over 75 per cent;
- engaging 4,00,000 female Accredited Social Health Activists (ASHAs).

The deviation from the stated objectives and measured outcomes is glaring in the case of NCDs. Though included in the objectives, there was no programmatic emphasis on that large and growing public health problem, nor was there an attempt to affix measurable targets to be achieved in this area. Perhaps, the erroneous impression that NCDs were mainly a problem in the urban areas and of the affluent led to an exclusive focus on maternal and child mortality, and infectious diseases, which are problems that afflict the poor disproportionately.

The fact remains that the NRHM became a selective health programme, focusing almost exclusively on maternal and child health, and infectious diseases. While the priority accorded to these was unexceptionable, it meant that many other health needs of the community were not addressed. This was contrary to the spirit of 'comprehensive primary healthcare' and reflected the 'selective primary healthcare' approach favoured by many international funders and reinforced by the MDGs. Consequently, the health system was fragmented by a disease-centric approach and segmented by an age-specific approach. Children under 5 and pregnant women became the focus of attention, while adolescents and the elderly especially lost out on services under the NRHM. Infectious diseases were included, but NCDs, mental health, injuries and snakebites, eye care, oral health, and several other areas did not feature under the NRHM.

Eighteen states with worse health indicators than others were chosen for special attention and placed under the label of 'Empowered Action Group' (EAG). The programme was extended to other states as well, but the EAG states were considered critical because of the commitment to reduce health gaps between states and also because these states weighed heavily on the aggregate national indicators targeted by the mission. An urban component was to be added to the rural mission later in 2013, with the conjoint programme being relabelled as the National Health Mission (NHM).

The mission proposed several important health system-strengthening features. These included: the introduction of village-level community mobilisers in the form of ASHAs; strengthening of infrastructure in the primary healthcare facility chain, from sub-centres to community health centres; introduction of demand-side financial incentives for stimulating people to seek health services and utilise health facilities; decentralisation of health planning up to the district level; greater devolution of financial powers to states and districts; increased engagement of the communities and Panchayati Raj institutions in the implementation and strengthening of health management information systems.

The most visible, and perhaps the most useful, innovation brought by the NRHM to the health system is the introduction of the ASHA. A locally resident village woman (married, divorced or widowed), in the age group of 25–45 years and with a class 8 education, initially acted as the mobiliser for institutional deliveries and child immunisation. She received performance-based financial incentives for those. In recent years, tasks and incentives have also been added on—from programmes related to infectious diseases, family planning, adolescent health, water, sanitation and nutrition. She is also expected to provide health education to the community and serves as a depot holder for oral rehydration therapy, iron and folic acid tablets, chloroquine, condoms and oral contraceptive pills. Over 9,00,000 ASHAS now mark the march of the NRHM across the country. Despite their increasing role, the ASHAs are still assigned a volunteer status and not recognised as a regular part of the organised health services. This stems from a bureaucratic apprehension that formally linking them to the health workforce may lead to their getting 'unionised' and becoming less efficient!

The devolution of the financial powers to district-level societies was definitely a democratic step, as was the intended bottom-up approach to the development of district- and state-level Project Implementation Plans. Despite the promised devolution, it has taken a while for the rigid bureaucratic channels to relax their centralised controls. Nevertheless, the design feature is laudable. Similarly, the emphasis on community engagement and the formation of Rogi Kalyan Samitis was forward-looking. The expected engagement of Panchayat Raj institutions, however, remained at a low ebb. Health information systems improved and the annual Common Review Missions provided for evaluation by independent experts.

The mission did have partial success. It increased the proportion of deliveries that were conducted in healthcare facilities ('institutional deliveries') as compared to those that happened at home. This was partly because of the role played by the ASHAs and the financial incentives provided both to the ASHAs and to the pregnant women. No clear correlation was demonstrable between the rise in institutional deliveries spurred by the financial incentives and the decline in maternal mortality, raising questions about the quality of care at the institutions which conducted the deliveries (Randive, Diwan and De Costa 2013). However, the secular trend in the decline of maternal mortality accelerated after the launch of the NRHM (Figure 5.1). While the initial targets of the NRHM were not achieved in the specified timelines and India also did not achieve the MDG targets by 2015, maternal mortality fell to 130 in 2014–16 from 167 in 2011–13 (Ministry of Health and Family Welfare 2017). This rate of decline is higher than the global average during this period and sets the pace for reaching the SDG target of 70 by 2030. It appears that some further acceleration, however, would be needed.

Engagement of the states in the mission was variable in extent and impact. Some of the EAG states improved in their performance, while others failed to utilise the mission adequately

Figure 5.1: Trends in MMR in India

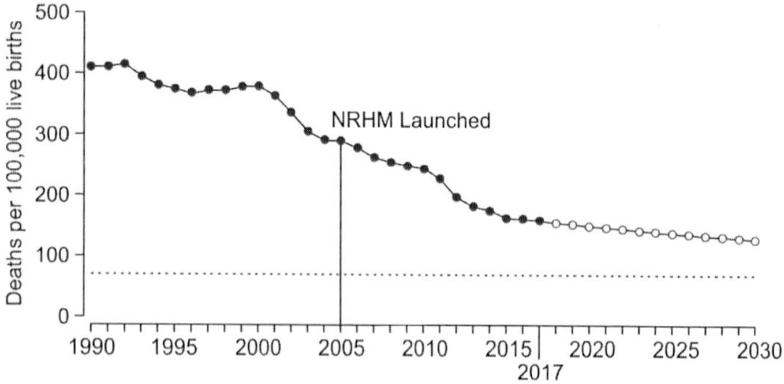

Source: Adapted by author from Vos et al. 2017 and additional data accessed from The Global Burden of Disease study (provided by the Institute of Health Metrics and Evaluation).

because of poor governance. Lack of adequate numbers of skilled human resources at various levels of healthcare has been a major impediment that limited the impact of the NRHM. Transport services for health emergencies became more widely available. However, static primary healthcare facilities in some states still faced problems of uncertain electricity and water supplies. The urban component of the expanded mission has remained on the anvil far too long and has not adapted well to the distinct needs of urban primary healthcare.

While the NRHM had several deficiencies in design and execution, it infused a sense of purpose into the health system. It provided a platform for concerted engagement of state and central agencies, while creating space for inter-sectoral coordination. It offers the scope for the creation of a framework of comprehensive primary healthcare. In the first decade of the programme, the NRHM/NHM did not meet the needs of UHC, but can now be modified to fit into the UHC framework.

The Rashtriya Swasthya Bima Yojana

This central government-subsidised health insurance scheme was rolled out from 1 April 2008. Social security for the large number of informal workers became an important priority following the Arjun Sengupta Committee report on the informal workforce (National Commission for Enterprises in the Unorganised Sector 2007). Following the German model of social health insurance for workers, which marked the beginnings of the movement towards UHC in nineteenth-century Europe, the Ministry of Labour launched the RSBY in India. It was later transferred to the Health Ministry in 2015 (Government of India n.d.).

The scheme aimed to provide cashless healthcare to informal (unrecognised) workers who were below the poverty line. With a subscription of Rs 30 (US 45 cents), a family of five could expect annual coverage up to Rs 30,000 (USD 450). This was restricted to costs of care during hospitalisation and was administered through insurance companies. Both public and private hospitals were empanelled. Since the cost coverage was capped at Rs 30,000, the treatments were mostly restricted to secondary care and did not cover costly tertiary care. The costs of outpatient care and of medicines outside the hospital were not covered.

The scheme did increase access of the poor to some forms of hospitalised care. Initially, there were serious concerns about fraud, but fairly robust systems for fraud prevention and detection were created in response. However, the problem of induced demand continued to fester, with reports of unnecessary hysterectomies and cardiac procedures. Information technology was used to create a strong administrative backbone. Over time, the categories of beneficiaries were expanded to include other vulnerable groups. By 2017, the number of potential beneficiaries enrolled reached close to 3,00,000.

Not all states accepted this central scheme. Some of them were operating schemes of their own, often with distinctive political branding. The coverage cap was five to 10 times higher than provided by the RSBY, since the intent was to cover tertiary care, which was virtually inaccessible to the poor. In fact, the Rajiv Arogyasri scheme in Andhra Pradesh antedated the RSBY and the chief minister who introduced the scheme credited its popularity for his re-election. No wonder, then, that some other states, too, started their own versions of that programme. Some states wished to reserve the common procedures paid for by their schemes only to public hospitals to ensure that public funding would not mostly flow to private hospitals, weakening the public institutions further. However, the administrators of the RSBY did not permit such differentiation.

While the RSBY succeeded in increasing access to health services, it failed to provide the poor with the financial protection that was its major objective. This was revealed in several evaluations that were done. The principal reasons were the limited coverage cap, which often fell below the charges that the hospitals levied, and the failure to cover the post-hospitalisation costs incurred on outpatient care and medicines. This problem was noted also with the state insurance schemes, where tertiary care and long-term follow up care extracted high costs both within and outside the hospital. A report by Brookings India, which compared the findings of the National Sample Surveys of 2004 and 2014, reported that financial protection was not evident when assessed by any of three indicators (out-of-pocket healthcare expenditure; catastrophic healthcare expenditure; and healthcare-induced impoverishment). Indeed, the proportion of the Indian population that suffered healthcare-related poverty was 7 per cent in both 2004 and 2014 (Ravi, Ahluwalia and Bergkevist 2016).

Despite these disappointments, the RSBY helped to create a platform for increasing healthcare access to the poor through financial coverage of hospitalisation costs through a heavily government-subsidised insurance programme. It engaged the private sector in the delivery of services, though it could not fully prevent excesses by its errant sections. It built strong information technology-enabled administrative platforms. It has thereby provided the base for a more efficient and equitable cost coverage programme that may evolve under a future UHC framework. It was inadequate and, in some ways, inappropriate in its form and function, but could contribute its stronger elements to a new design.

References

Government of India. n.d. 'Rashtriya Swasthya Bima Yojana'. Available at https://www.india.gov.in/spotlight/rashtriya-swasthya-bima-yojana (accessed 28 November 2018).

Ministry of Health and Family Welfare. 2005. 'National Health Mission'. New Delhi. Available at http://nhm.gov.in/images/pdf/NHM/NHM_more_information.pdf (accessed 22 November 2018).

______. 2017. 'National Health Policy 2017'. New Delhi. Available at http://cdsco.nic.in/writereaddata/National-Health-Policy.pdf (accessed 22 November 2018).

National Commission for Enterprises in the Unorganised Sector. 2007. 'Report on Conditions of Work and Promotion of Livelihoods in the Unorganised Sector'. New Delhi. Available at http://dcmsme.gov.in/Condition_of_workers_sep_2007.pdf (accessed 22 November 2018).

NSSO. 2006. 'Household Consumer Expenditure' (NSS 61st Round: 2004–05). New Delhi.

Randive, B., V. Diwan, and A. De Costa. 2013. 'India's Conditional Cash Transfer Programme (the JSY) to Promote Institutional Birth: Is There an Association between Institutional Birth Proportion and Maternal Mortality?' *PLoS One* 8 (6): e67452.

Ravi, S., R. Ahluwalia, and S. Bergkevist. 2016. 'Health and Morbidity in India (2004–2014)'. New Delhi. Available at https://www.brookings.edu/wp-content/uploads/2016/12/201612_health-and-morbidity.pdf (accessed 28 November 2018).

Vos, T., A. A. Abajobir, C. Abbafati, K. M. Abbas, K. H. Abate, F. Abd-Allah, et al. 2017. 'Global, Regional, and National Incidence, Prevalence, and Years Lived with Disability for 328 Diseases and Injuries for 195 Countries, 1990–2016: A Systematic Analysis for the Global Burden of Disease Study 2016'. *Lancet* 390 (10100): P1211–59.

World Health Organization. 2008. 'The World Health Report 2008—Primary Health Care (Now More Than Ever)'. Geneva. Available at https://www.who.int/whr/2008/en/ (accessed 22 February 2019).

six

The High Level Expert Group

Providing a Framework for Universal Health Coverage

> The best form of providing health protection would be to change the economic system which produces ill health, and to liquidate ignorance, poverty and unemployment. The practice of each individual purchasing his own medical care does not work. It is unjust, inefficient, wasteful and completely outmoded ... In our highly geared, modern industrial society, there is no such thing as private health—all health is public. The illness and maladjustments of one unit of the mass affects all other members. The protection of people's health should be recognised by the Government as its primary obligation and duty to its citizens.
>
> Norman Bethune, 1936 (Allan and Gordon 1952)

The Genesis

While the NRHM and the RSBY served to improve access to some health services, they were a far cry from comprehensive primary healthcare and UHC. Services in the NRHM were mostly focussed on maternal and child health. Major public health challenges like NCDs and disorders of mental health were not addressed. Quality of care was sub-optimal in many states due to severe shortages in qualified health personnel. The RSBY, too, provided limited financial coverage for hospitalisation at the secondary care level and did not cover outpatient care, which accounted for the largest fraction of impoverishing out-of-pocket expenditure. By 2010, the call for UHC began to get amplified at both national and global levels, with the publication of the World Health Report that year, entitled 'Health Systems Financing: Road To Universal Health Coverage'. Dr Manmohan Singh, then Prime Minister of India, advised the Planning Commission of India to design a framework for UHC.

A High Level Expert Group (HLEG) on UHC was constituted by the Planning Commission in October 2010, with the mandate of developing a framework for providing easily accessible and affordable healthcare to all Indians (Planning Commission 2011). While financial protection was the principal objective of this initiative, it was recognised that the delivery of UHC also requires availability of adequate healthcare infrastructure, skilled health workforce, and access to affordable drugs and technologies to ensure the entitled level and quality of care to every citizen. Further, the design and delivery of health programmes and services call for efficient management systems and active engagement of empowered communities. The original terms of reference directed the HLEG to address all of these needs of UHC. Since the social determinants of health have a profound influence not only on the health of populations but also on the ability of individuals to access healthcare, the HLEG decided to include a clear reference to them, though such determinants are conventionally regarded as falling in the domain of non-health sectors.

The HLEG's Vision

The HLEG's vision of UHC transcended the narrow, inadequate and often inequitable view of UHC as merely a system of health insurance. UHC, in its understanding, moves beyond 'insurance' by providing an 'assurance' of healthcare for multiple needs and includes health beyond healthcare, not being confined to a mere illness response. The HLEG affirmed that UHC should address health in all of its dimensions and emphasise prevention and primary healthcare, which are ignored, neglected or even undermined by the usual systems of health insurance. Such an assurance of health in all dimensions has to be provided by the government, which has to act as the guarantor of UHC and ensure its success and sustainability by mobilising all societal resources and advance multi-sectoral actions. In this perspective of the HLEG, UHC is linked firmly to the Right to Health and converts an aspirational goal into an entitled provision.

The HLEG sought to unambiguously state this vision it chose for UHC. This was especially needed in view of the prevalent (and still ongoing) debates on Universal Health Coverage versus Universal Health Care. Proponents of the latter were of the view that coverage was limited to enrolment under a scheme, usually under a health insurance programme, and offered no assurance of adequate and appropriate service provision at an affordable cost. However, coverage was used by others to include all of those elements. Since Universal Health Coverage was adopted as a goal by the World Health Assembly in 2005, the HLEG adhered to that terminology of UHC, but took care to explicitly define what was meant.

HLEG's Definition on UHC

'Ensuring equitable access for all Indian citizens, resident in any part of the country, regardless of income level, social status, gender, caste or religion, to affordable, accountable, appropriate health services of assured quality (promotive, preventive, curative and rehabilitative)

as well as public health services addressing the wider determinants of health delivered to individuals and populations, with the government being the guarantor and enabler, although not necessarily the only provider, of health and related services' (Planning Commission 2011).

This definition incorporated the different dimensions of universal health assurance: *healthcare*, which includes ensuring access to a wide range of promotive, preventive, curative, and rehabilitative health services at different levels of care; *health coverage*, which is inclusive of all sections of the population; and *health protection*, which promotes and protects health through its social determinants. These services should be delivered at an affordable cost, so that people do not suffer financial hardship in the pursuit of good health.

The HLEG asserted that the foundation for UHC is a universal entitlement to comprehensive health security and an all-encompassing obligation on the part of the state (the government) to provide adequate food and nutrition, appropriate medical care, access to safe drinking water, proper sanitation, education, health-related information and other contributors to good health. It was the HLEG's stated belief that the state should be primarily and principally responsible for ensuring and guaranteeing UHC for its citizens. The state should not only provide health and related services, but should also address the wider determinants of health to effectively guarantee health security.

Guiding Principles of UHC

Ten principles guided the formulation of the HLEG's recommendations for introducing a system of UHC in India: (i) universality; (ii) equity; (iii) non-exclusion and non-discrimination; (iv) comprehensive care that is rational and of good quality; (v) financial protection; (vi) protection of patients' rights that guarantee appropriateness of care, patient choice, portability and continuity of care; (vii) consolidated and strengthened public health provisioning; (viii) accountability and transparency; (ix) community participation; and (x) putting health in people's hands (Planning Commission 2011).

Intrinsic to the notion of universality, non-discrimination, non-exclusion and equity is a fundamental commitment to health as a human right. Universality implies that no one (especially marginalised, remote and migrant communities as well as communities that have been historically discriminated against) is excluded from a system of UHC. At the same time, while society should pay special attention to the concerns of disadvantaged populations and the poor, a universal system should provide health coverage and care for everyone. This will ensure the creation of a robust and sustainable system of UHC in whose success every section of society has a vital interest. It will also protect both the poor and non-poor from the risk of impoverishment due to unaffordable healthcare expenditures. The HLEG was of the view that any system of UHC can succeed only if it is established on the strong foundations of common interest, social solidarity and cross-subsidisation.

The HLEG's report states that a system of UHC for India requires a flexible architecture to deal with inequities in health outcomes, regional and socio-cultural diversity, and the differential healthcare needs of populations in different locations. It should also take into account the challenges of rapid urbanisation, simultaneous demographic, epidemiological and nutritional transitions underway, and also social and political changes occurring in the country.

Embedded in the report's understanding of UHC is the recognition of two critical factors. First, it will be difficult, if not impossible, to achieve and sustain UHC without addressing the social determinants of health. Urgent and concrete actions addressing the social determinants of health are needed to move towards greater health equity, bridge gaps and reduce differentials in health by class, caste, gender and region across the country. In other words, UHC can be achieved only when sufficient and simultaneous attention is paid to: nutrition and food security, water and sanitation, social inclusion to address concerns of gender, caste, religious and tribal minorities, decent housing, a clean environment, employment and work security, occupational safety and disaster management. Second, the very framework and principles of UHC for India will be severely undermined if gender insensitivity and gender discrimination remain unaddressed. An inclusive approach to health should attend to the needs and differentials between men, women and other genders, along with the interaction between social and biological markers of health. For making UHC truly gender-sensitive, HLEG specifically recommended critical actions to improve access for women and girls to health services (going beyond maternal and child health), to recognise and strengthen women's central role in healthcare provision in both the formal health system and in the home, to build up the capacity of the health system to recognise, measure, monitor and address gender concerns, and to support and empower girls and women.

Based on a review of the global experience with UHC leads, the HLEG concluded that there does not appear to be a single universal method of financing and financial protection that assures guaranteed UHC in any country. Therefore, what the report proposed for India was a somewhat unique hybrid system that draws on the lessons learned from India and from other developed and developing countries.

The HLEG's vision and recommendations took cognisance of the extraordinary opportunities that India offers—and the possibility for India to take a lead in introducing a well-designed UHC system that is eminently suited to the needs and resources of countries at a similar level of development. The path forward was clearly delineated:

> We propose that every citizen should be entitled to essential primary, secondary and tertiary health care services that will be guaranteed by the Central government. The range of essential health care services offered as a National Health Package (NHP) will cover all common conditions and high-impact, cost-effective health care interventions for reducing health-related mortality and disability. A panel of experts should determine the package of services taking into account the resource availability as well as the health care needs of the country. Health care services to all citizens covered under UHC will be made available through the public sector and contracted-in private facilities (including non-governmental organisations [NGOs] and non-profits) (Planning Commission 2011).

Key Recommendations of the HLEG Report

1. The central and state governments combined should increase the public expenditures on health from 1.2 per cent (in 2010) to at least 2.5 per cent (by 2017) and to at least 3 per cent (by 2022) of the nation's GDP. Thus, two five-year plan periods were to be covered from 2012 to step up public financing substantially to meet the needs of UHC.

   This was expected to reduce private out-of-pocket spending from 67 per cent (in 2010) to 33 per cent (by 2022). The case for increased public financing, as an essential ingredient for successful delivery of UHC, was clearly made in the report citing global evidence and highlighting the consequences of low public financing.

2. Use general taxation as the principal source of healthcare financing, complemented by additional mandatory deductions for healthcare from salaried individuals and tax payers, either as a proportion of taxable income or as a proportion of salary.

   Since success of UHC is dependent on a high level of public financing, especially in India, with a large segment of the population poor and the vast majority of the workforce operating in the informal sector, the HLEG considered a tax-funded model of UHC as the best suited for the country.

3. Expenditures on primary healthcare, including general health information and promotion, curative services at the primary level and cost-effective treatment, targeted towards specific risk factors, should account for at least 70 per cent of all healthcare expenditures.

   Primary healthcare provides the foundation for UHC, because every person needs services provided at that level sometime or other in life. Primary health services are, therefore, truly universal in coverage. They cater to common health problems faced by the people. While providing the platform for a wide range of preventive services, primary healthcare catalyses and facilitates health promotion initiatives in the community. By enabling early detection and timely treatment for a number of disorders, it can slow down their progression, thereby preventing complications that demand expensive advanced care. Primary care also acts as a responsible gatekeeper for referral to secondary and tertiary care, while receiving people back from those levels for follow-up care. It is the best setting for providing chronic continuous care for conditions like hypertension and diabetes, while ensuring close to home antenatal care during pregnancy. However, primary healthcare has long been neglected in health financing as resources have flowed preferentially to hospitals providing advanced care to fewer numbers of people. This has happened both through direct funding and through government-sponsored health insurance schemes. The HLEG called for correction of this anomaly.

4. All government-funded health insurance schemes should be, over time, integrated with the UHC system. The RSBY should be transferred from the Ministry of Labour to the Ministry of Health and Family Welfare and the technical and other capacities developed by the RSBY should be utilised for the operations of UHC.

The fragmentation of public financing across multiple government-sponsored health insurance schemes promotes redundancy, reduces purchasing power and hinders portability of financial protection across the country. This is especially so when central- and state-sponsored schemes compete with each other. Merging these schemes expands the resource pool and enlarges the risk pool, permitting a larger package of services under UHC.

The RSBY was set up under the Labour Ministry, following the original German model of social protection for workers. The large number of informal workers in India stimulated such a scheme which was designed and operated by the Labour Ministry. However, the health systems through which the health services are to be provided under the scheme are governed by the central and state governments. For reasons of efficiency and economy, the scheme has to function in conjunction with the other health services offered by these governments. Therefore, it was considered operationally appropriate to transfer the RSBY to the Health Ministry. Merger of all government-funded schemes, with progressive integration of employer-funded insurance schemes, would lead to the creation of a single payer system which makes the purchasing of services much more efficient and economical.

5. Governments or quasi-governmental agencies must purchase health services under the UHC system. That function should not be entrusted to insurance companies.

The HLEG recognised that, in India's mixed health system, direct provision of health services by the government would need to be supplemented by the contracted services provided by the private sector (including the not-for-profit healthcare providers). However, it was of the view that the purchasing of services for UHC should be a function of empowered government departments or quasi-governmental autonomous bodies established by and accountable to the government. The functioning of the existing central- and state-funded health insurance schemes had yielded experience of both insurance companies and government established trusts acting as the purchasing intermediaries. Despite the expertise available in insurance companies for handling traditional insurance products, they were considered a misfit for handling public finances for UHC. This was partly due to high overhead costs and escalating premiums, but, more importantly, because of their lack of commitment to a public sector-led, primary care-prioritised design of UHC wherein primary care services and public sector hospitals would need to be progressively strengthened. A single-payer system also argued against multiple insurance intermediaries.

6. No user fee should be levied at the point of care. All health services under UHC must be pre-paid and provided free at the time of care.

   While user fee was advocated by global financing institutions such as the World Bank before the turn of the twentieth century, global experience clearly demonstrated that user fee was inefficient, inadequate and inequitable. It was inefficient because of the cumbersome collection systems that involved dedicated clerical work for collection, time delays in getting care, and stress caused to patients and families in negotiating the payment system. It was inadequate because the fee collected in public facilities was often insufficient and needed substantial supplementation from tax revenues. Most important, it was inequitable as evidence showed that even small amounts of user fee shut the doors on the poor and reduced their access to needed healthcare. The HLEG, therefore, called for a pre-paid system which did not demand user fee from the patient at the point of care but would pay the provider through the price negotiated purchasing mechanism of UHC.

7. Public financing must be used to provide essential drugs free of cost.

   The largest fraction of out-of-pocket expenditure on healthcare arises from spending on medicines. If essential medicines are unaffordable, adherence to life-saving treatments becomes irregular or abandoned. If people do purchase despite the financial difficulties, there is a danger of being pushed into poverty, especially if the treatment needed is lifelong or long-term. To obviate these undesirable outcomes, essential drugs must be provided free of cost. The HLEG estimated that this can be done at a relatively low cost to public funding, at around 0.5 per cent of the GDP. This can provide early and substantial relief to people, even as UHC evolves in stages.

8. Develop a National Health Package, with flexibility for incorporating state-specific requirements, listing entitled health services at every level of the healthcare delivery system. Reorient healthcare provision to focus significantly on primary healthcare.

   Such a package would take into account the healthcare needs of the population and the resources available. Timely preventive, promotive, diagnostic, curative and rehabilitative services should be provided at appropriate levels of healthcare delivery. Five levels of care were identified by the HLEG; the first three focused on primary healthcare at sub-centre, primary health centre and community health centre levels. The other two related to secondary and tertiary care at more advanced facilities. Well-functioning primary healthcare teams, apart from providing timely and cost-effective care, can also potentially promote health equity by improving social cohesion, reducing discrimination, and empowering communities to improve their health conditions.

9. Strengthen district hospitals.

   The HLEG advocated strengthening of district hospitals, with adequate equipment and suitable staffing. The district hospital has a critical role to play in healthcare delivery and health professional training under the UHC system, both of which should be well attuned to the needs of the particular district, while conforming to national standards of healthcare provision. A well-resourced primary healthcare system, supported by a strengthened district hospital which is backed as needed by a contracting of effectively regulated private hospitals, should aim to meet 95 per cent of the healthcare needs of the district.

10. Develop effective contracting-in guidelines, with adequate checks and balances, for the provision of healthcare by the formal private sector.

    Recognising that India's mixed health system has to optimally utilise all sectors therein for effective service delivery under UHC, the report recommended a shift from a potpourri of poorly designed PPPs to a well-defined service delivery partnership between the government as a purchaser and the private sector as a provider. Thereby, the government would engage the not-for-profit and for-profit private sector, and also frontline NGOs, to supplement the services provided by the public sector. This would require (i) a strong regulation, accreditation and supervisory framework based on state-level decision-making on the degree of UHC provision by each contracted private institution (which must dedicate at least 75 per cent of outpatient and 50 per cent of inpatient services within its healthcare facility); (ii) control of the manner in which various inputs are deployed by the provider; (iii) careful tracking of both immediate and longer-term outcomes; and (iv) a specifically designated population group to be served by the provider.

11. Ensure equitable access to functional beds for guaranteeing secondary and tertiary care.

    The report recommended an increase in functional bed capacity to at least two hospital beds per 1,000 of the population by 2022. It emphasised the need for equitable distribution so that a sufficient number of functional beds are available in small towns and rural areas, as opposed to prevailing urban concentration.

12. Reorganise urban healthcare for efficiency and equity, focusing particularly on the health needs of the urban poor.

    The HLEG recommended a new urban UHC system that offers a defined package of services at each level through clearly designated primary, secondary and tertiary care facilities. The efficiency of the public health system in urban areas should be strengthened by improving urban primary health services, healthcare infrastructure and designated referral facilities. Deployment of nurse practitioners and engagement of communities through urban local bodies would strengthen urban primary care. Particular attention would be needed to be paid to the health needs of persons in low-income urban communities.

13. Ensure adequate number of trained healthcare providers and technical healthcare workers at different levels by: (i) giving primacy to the provision of primary healthcare; and (ii) increasing HRH density to achieve WHO norms of at least 23 health workers per 10,000 of the population (doctors, nurses and midwives).

    Specifically, the HLEG recommended the doubling of community health workers (ASHAs) to two per 1,000 of the population, introduction of a new three-year Bachelor of Rural Health Care (BRHC) degree programme, an increase in the availability of nurses to 1.7 million by 2017 and 2.7 million by 2022, increase in the production of allopathic doctors to reach a ratio of one per 1,000 of the population by 2027, active engagement of AYUSH doctors in primary healthcare and equitable deployment of allied health professionals across the country.

14. Invest in additional educational institutions to produce and train the requisite health workforce, while enhancing

the quality of education and training by introducing competency-based, health system-connected curricula and continuous education.

The report proposed setting up of new nursing and medical colleges in districts with little or no presence of such colleges and setting up of new ANM schools in states which have insufficient capacity to reach the target norm of two ANMs per sub-health centre. It emphasised that curricula in health professional training colleges must keep pace with the changing dynamics of public health, health policy and health demographics. Greater priority should be accorded to population-based primary and preventive care, in health professional education.

15. Establish District Health Knowledge Institutes.

Alongside strengthening district hospitals for better healthcare delivery, they can also support health professional training for all health, family planning and nutrition programmes operating in that district. The HLEG proposed the establishment of District Health Knowledge Training Institutes, which are autonomous but operationally affiliated to the district hospital. The BRHC courses too should run from there. The report recommended that districts serving more than 5,00,000 persons must initially establish such institutes which should also establish connectivity with locally situated medical and nursing colleges.

16. Establish a National Council for Human Resources in Health.

The proposed council would prescribe, monitor and promote standards of health professional education. It was envisaged to be a body that would provide overarching regulation of competency-based medical, dental, nursing, pharmacy, public health and allied health professional education and serve as a platform for promoting inter-professional education.

17. Increase access to drugs through higher public expenditure, price control on essential drugs and pooled public procurement.

    An early measure to substantially reduce out-of-pocket expenditure is to provide essential drugs free of cost in public facilities. While this will entail higher public expenditure, the HLEG estimated that it could be done by allocating 0.5 per cent of the GDP for this purpose. Pooled public procurement would also enable the government to lower the cost of purchase. Both allopathic and AYUSH drugs could be purchased through this mechanism. Price controls on essential drugs are also recommended to ensure affordability.

18. Ensure drug and vaccine security by strengthening the public sector capacity for production, protecting domestic private sector manufacturing capacity and safeguarding the flexibility provided by the TRIPS agreement.

    Expanding and strengthening domestic capacity for drug and vaccine manufacture, in both public and private sectors, is essential to have assured access to medicines and vaccines at affordable prices. The ability to manufacture generics and utilise the flexibility, offered by the TRIPS agreement, should not be compromised by foreign acquisition of Indian firms or by free trade agreements, which obstruct compulsory licensing and impose data exclusivity clauses.

19. Set up national and state drug supply logistics corporations.

    The report recommended the establishment of autonomous corporations for bulk procurement of low-cost, generic, essential drugs. The Tamil Nadu model was considered as an example of an effective, transparent and adaptable public procurement system. It was also recommended that there should be at least one warehouse in each district to ensure availability of drugs to all providers, with information technology-enabled tracking to avoid stock-outs and interruptions in supply.

20. Promote community participation and citizen engagement by transforming existing Village Health Committees into participatory Health Councils and organising regular Health Assemblies.

    Since community empowerment and active engagement are essential for the success of UHC, the report recommended that the models developed in Brazil and Thailand be adopted to increase citizen participation in priority-setting processes and monitoring. The existing Village Health and Sanitation Committees should be transformed to decision-making Health Councils and an annual Health Assembly should be organised at state and national levels, with citizen participation. This would lead to democratisation of the health system and bring citizen support to UHC.

21. Strengthen the role of elected representatives, local bodies, civil society and NGOs.

    Local planning for health service delivery under UHC and monitoring of its implementation would require the empowered participation of Panchayat Raj institutions and elected urban municipal bodies. While the NRHM has incorporated the engagement of Panchayat Raj institutions in its design, the operational plans do not accord an active role for them. The urban local bodies are even more distanced due to the non-commencement of an urban health mission. These disconnects need to be addressed, if UHC has to draw upon the strength of local leadership.

22. Establish all-India and state-level Public Health Service Cadres and a specialised state-level Health Systems Management Cadre in order to give greater attention to public health and also to strengthen the management of the UHC system.

    Public health expertise is required for the health promotion and prevention components of UHC, and for design, implementation and monitoring of the health system strengthening initiatives needed for the success of UHC. Multidisciplinary public health learning is missing in the health systems of the country and public health expertise is not utilised to advance planning and delivery of health programmes. Tamil Nadu, the only exception, has demonstrated the value of a dedicated public health cadre in improving the implementation of health programmes, and in the organisation of primary and secondary health services. A defined Public Health Cadre at central and state levels was, therefore, recommended by the HLEG.

23. Develop a national health information technology network based on uniform standards, to ensure interoperability between all healthcare stakeholders.

    Prioritisation, delivery and monitoring of services under UHC will require a strong information technology platform. This needs to connect all levels of the health system and the agencies managing UHC. Portability of UHC benefits will also require connectivity across all regions of the country. The report emphasises the need to establish such a network to serve the needs of UHC.

24. Establish several regulatory agencies: National Health Regulatory and Development Authority (NHRDA); National

Drug Regulatory and Development Authority (NDRDA); and National Health Promotion and Protective Trust (NHPPT).

Design and delivery of UHC calls for stronger and more efficiently organised regulatory architecture than was seen in the prevailing health system. The HLEG called for the establishment of a national body, the NHRDA, to perform the various functions needed for designing and managing UHC (Figure 1.1). The NHRDA will have a System Support Unit, a National Health and Medical Facilities Accreditation Unit and a Health Evaluation Unit. The NHRDA would have state-level counterparts (SHRDAs) which would perform several of those functions at the state level while coordinating with NHRDA.

25. Adopt better human resource practices to improve recruitment, retention motivation and performance; rationalise pay and incentives and assure career tracks for competency-based professional advancement.

    The HLEG recognised that shortages in the health workforce were aggravated by poor governance and cadre management practices in the health system. Arbitrary postings and transfers, poor pay scales and lack of career advancement opportunities are demotivating factors for many categories of health workers. The report called for better human resource management practices to improve recruitment and retention in the public sector.

Expected Outcomes from UHC

The HLEG concluded its case for UHC in India by summarising the benefits that can be expected if the country adopts and implements it in earnest.

India can aspire to achieve greater equity by bridging health disparities and inequities. The creation of a strong and robust health policy platform through the proposed scaling up of public spending and expansion in health service provisioning is likely to improve health outcomes. Moreover, the adoption of an integrated primary health approach is expected to result in a gradual but significant reduction in overall disease burden across the country. A strengthened health system under UHC will result in better health literacy for Indians through improved health promotion, healthier behaviours and lifestyles. Greater emphasis on the use of information technology to link health care networks will improve health surveillance in the country with the establishment of a health information system that will generate valuable data on various health and disease trends and outcomes.

The expansion of the health workforce is also expected to generate almost seven million jobs for young people and women over the coming decade. The provision of pre-paid health services and free medicines for both inpatient as well as outpatient care can be expected to significantly reduce the high private out of pocket spending. A healthy population in turn can contribute to economic growth through increased productivity and higher earnings. There are other benefits as well. Promoting health equity also contributes to increased social cohesion and empowerment and by joining the global movement towards UHC India now has both the capacity and opportunity to emerge as leading force for equitable health care of all. And finally, through implementing UHC with its unique reach and scope of health care delivery, India stands to gain the political goodwill and support of 1.2 billion potential beneficiaries (Planning Commission 2011).

The Aftermath

The HLEG report was widely debated in the central government and the civil society. The Ministry of Health and Family Welfare did not identify with the report because it viewed it as an initiative of the Planning Commission, even though the Mission Director of the NRHM (an Additional Secretary in the Ministry) was a member of the HLEG. According to newspaper reports of the day, the Prime Minister's office was briefed that the report was too radical and its implementation would need an extensive overhaul of the existing system. Neither the Health Ministry nor the Planning Commission engaged the states in a discussion on the report. The national consensus that was needed to make UHC politically viable and operationally feasible was not even attempted by either of these agencies, which ideally should have steered those consultations.

The civil society largely welcomed the report, though one section expressed concerns about engaging the private sector for publicly funded service delivery under UHC. This was despite the caveats and the regulatory measures proposed in the report to carefully contract and manage the private sector in a supplementary gap-filling role as needed in the existing mixed health system. In light of the much greater leeway given to the private sector in later health reforms in India, this criticism of the HLEG report appears to have been unduly suspicious of even the circumscribed role envisaged for that sector in the HLEG's report. In retrospect, a valuable opportunity was lost for uniting the civil society in a strong call for adoption and implementation of the HLEG report. The private sector itself was not enthused by a report which called for strengthening of the public sector and stricter regulation of the private sector.

The Planning Commission of India did allude to the HLEG report in its twelfth Five Year Plan (Planning Commission 2013). This document proposed to raise health expenditure to 1.87 per cent of the GDP by 2017. It also proposed piloting of UHC in one to two districts in each state during the plan period, to provide learnings from different models for informing the design for UHC scale up in the next plan. The responsibility for working with the states to initiate this effort and fund the pilots was given to the health ministry, which did not evince interest in pursuing it. Similarly, the twelfth Plan recommendation to create Public Health and Health Management Cadres in the states was also not pursued seriously by the Health Ministry.

At the political level, there was great commitment to the enactment of the Food Security Act before the elections of 2014. While this was a worthy cause deserving of political championing, health remained on the edge of the policy radar. It appeared the government was satisfied it had done enough through the NRHM and the RSBY and felt that further reforms in health could be examined after the elections of May 2014. As it happened, the government which initiated the HLEG report and then put it in cold storage yielded place to another national government in that election. It was now left to the new government to re-examine UHC through its own reform agenda.

References

Allan, T., and S. Gordon. 1952. *The Scalpel, the Sword: The Story of Doctor Norman Bethune*, ed. M. Carroll. Toronto: Dundurn Press.

Planning Commission. 2011. 'High Level Expert Group Report on Universal Health Coverage for India'. New Delhi. Available at https://docs.google.com/viewer?url=http://planningcommission.nic.in/reports/genrep/rep_uhc0812.pdf (accessed 12 November 2018).

———. 2013. 'Twelfth Five Year Plan (2012–2017); Social Sectors'. New Delhi. Available at http://planningcommission.gov.in/plans/planrel/12thplan/welcome.html (accessed 12 November 2018).

seven

National Health Policy 2017

> Improve health status through concerted policy action in all sectors and expand preventive, promotive, curative, palliative and rehabilitative services provided through the public health sector with focus on quality.
>
> National Health Policy 2017

Efforts to design a new National Health Policy (NHP) were initiated in 2014 (Ministry of Health and Family Welfare 2017), when a new government took power at the centre. The previous policy was of 2002 (Ministry of Health and Family Welfare 2003) vintage and much had changed in India's health profile and the health system responses, warranting a new policy to create the vision and vehicles for transforming the country's health over the next decade. A draft of the proposed NHP emerged into public view in 2015 (Ministry of Health and Family Welfare 2015), to be subjected to public comment and intra-governmental debates. Divergence in the perspectives of the Ministry of Health and Family Welfare and the government's think tank, the NITI Aayog, appeared to delay consensus on NHP. Finally, after a gestation period of two years, NHP 2017 was released in March 2017 (Ministry of Health and Family Welfare 2017).

The timing of the release of NHPs in 2002 and 2017 had resonance with major global developments led by the United Nations. NHP 2002 came two years after adoption of the MDGs

(WHO 2015). Similarly, NHP 2017 came two years after the adoption of the SDGs (United Nations Development Programme 2015). While India's NHPs essentially reflected the country's experience and aspirations, the vision was shaped partly by the global commitments made through the endorsement of MDGs and SDGs at different time periods.

NHP 2017 opens with a clearly stated goal that reflects the health goal of the SDGs, especially the commitment to UHC. The goal affirms:

> The policy envisages as its goal the attainment of the highest possible level of health and well-being for all at all ages, through a preventive and promotive health care orientation in all developmental policies, and universal access to good quality health care services without anyone having to face financial hardship as a consequence. This would be achieved through increasing access, improving quality and lowering the cost of healthcare delivery.
>
> The policy recognizes the pivotal importance of Sustainable Development Goals (SDGs). An indicative list of time bound quantitative goals aligned to ongoing national efforts as well as the global strategic directions is detailed (Ministry of Health and Family Welfare 2017).

While the vision is highly commendable, is this a rights-based assurance of UHC? In the transition between the draft and the final form, an important deletion was the reference to the intended enactment of the right to health. This omission has attracted criticism from the public health community and broader civil society on the grounds that the commitments made in the NHP can be guaranteed only if backed by such a right, in the absence of which expectations cannot translate to entitlements and assurances can remain undelivered. Apart from quibbling over what constitutes the right to health, it was the ambivalence over the government accepting a legal obligation to act as the guarantor that led to the retraction of this vital element in the final version of the NHP. In doing so, India failed to emulate the example of several developing countries, especially those in Latin America.

Nevertheless, NHP 2017 does set forth on a determined path of health system transformation that can lead to UHC, provided the policy is pursued with the correctives needed to remove the disconnects and distortions that deviate from the core principles of UHC. While espousing a strong public health approach and declaring a commitment to strengthening the public sector, the policy aims to draw upon the diverse systems of medicine practised in India and the different sectors of healthcare providers that form the ensemble cast of our mixed health system, for providing much-needed health services across India. In doing so, care must be taken to ensure that the role assigned to the private sector should not dilute the social commitment of the public sector. It must also be recognised that delinking of primary, secondary and tertiary care services, through separate financing and governance mechanisms, also poses a threat to the principle of primary healthcare-led UHC.

Although the need to establish inter-sectoral linkages to act on the varied social determinants of health is acknowledged by the policy, the content is mostly confined to aspirations and actions within the health sector. Unless the health sector exerts its influence on other sectors to sensitise them to public health at the policy level and convergence at the programme implementation level, health cannot be promoted or protected in all dimensions. Together, actions in the health sector and also in other health-relevant sectors can provide the blueprint for improving India's health, if implemented in earnest. The NHP does signal its intent to provide this broad sweep, though specific actions are not detailed.

The principal elements of NHP 2017 are as follows (Ministry of Health and Family Welfare 2017):

Increase in Public Financing

The policy acknowledges the need for raising the level of public financing for health and commits to raise it to 2.5 per cent of the GDP by 2025. This requires a doubling of the public expenditure on health in eight years. While this, too, is sub-optimal and projects a timeline that is farther than public health advocates had hoped for, it is still welcome as it promises to end several decades of low-level stagnation in public funding. For this to be credible, central and state budgets must reflect a steady and substantial annual rise. However, such a commitment was not visible in the budgets of 2018 and 2019. The policy also explicitly calls on the state governments to raise the proportion of budgetary allocation for health to above 8 per cent of their total budgets by 2020. Most states will need to double their health budgets in three years to reach this level. It remains to be seen as to what extent the states will respond to this directive.

Prioritisation of Primary Healthcare

Even as a case is made for increased public financing of health, NHP 2017 rightly affirms that 70 per cent of all such funding should go to primary healthcare, which is needed for comprehensive care and promotion of wellbeing. Continuity of care at the primary level and effective integration with other levels of care are envisaged. These services are to be available anywhere in the country, on the basis of a 'family card' that connects the family to a 'Health and Wellness Centre', which will emerge from the revamping of a primary care sub-centre. This centre will provide basic health services, referral linkages and perform a gatekeeper function for advanced care.

The delivery of the defined 'package of services' will be mostly through trained non-physician healthcare providers. Technology would be leveraged to provide bi-directional connectivity with higher levels of care.

Along with such strengthening of rural primary health services, the much-delayed National Urban Health Mission is also to be imparted with speed and scale to address the unmet needs of urban primary healthcare. This has been pending for a long time, despite the rising levels of urbanisation and unmet health needs of the urban poor. Lack of well-planned and dependable urban primary health services also results in flooding of secondary and tertiary care facilities with problems that could and should have been handled at the primary care level.

Strategic Purchasing of Secondary and Tertiary Care

While the policy mainly describes the role of the public sector in providing primary care, it is open about the intent to engage the private sector alongside the public sector, for the delivery of more advanced care at secondary and tertiary levels. There is a stated intent to strengthen district hospitals as well as sub-district hospitals and open more All-India Institutes of Medical Sciences in different regions, to augment public sector capacity for delivering advanced care. However, recognising the strong presence of the private sector at these levels, NHP 2017 proposes to undertake 'strategic purchasing' of secondary and tertiary healthcare services from both public and private sector healthcare facilities. Preference would be given to public, private non-profit and private for-profit hospitals, in that order. Given the erosion of public sector capacity over the years, 'strategic purchasing' may not provide a level playing field to the public sector to compete with the private sector. The disadvantaged public sector will steadily wither away, with the private sector capturing most of the public financing. With the public sector facilities marginalised, the private sector can dictate terms to the government in future purchasing transactions. Only a strong public sector, with committed government investment, can offer protection against such a dangerous tilt and provide the needed balance in our mixed health system.

Mode of Payment

While strategic purchasing has been indicated as the method by which the government will procure services from both public and private sectors, a distinction has been made in the mode of payment for primary healthcare and advanced healthcare. It has been proposed that a 'capitation' mode of payment will be adopted for primary healthcare and a 'fee for service' model would be adopted for secondary and tertiary care. The 'capitation' model refers to a fixed payment for a whole set of health services covering a person or a family in a year or any other defined period of time. This fixed sum would be paid to the healthcare provider to cover all healthcare costs incurred for a person in a year. While some of the individuals in the pool of persons registered for care under that provider will cross that coverage limit, many others will stay below the limit, making the scheme viable. More important, the provider has the incentive to focus on preventive and early care, to reduce the serious health conditions that demand costly advanced care. 'Fee for service', on the other hand, offers payment for each hospitalisation—indeed, for each medical consultation, procedure or test performed. This often becomes exorbitantly costly, by giving the provider a perverse incentive to perform more tests and procedures than necessary and call for more repeat specialist consultations than needed.

Surprisingly, the NHP disconnects primary from advanced care in the mode of payment. By restricting the 'capitation fee' model to primary care, the proposal strips the model of its ability to limit the costs of advanced care by incentivising provider commitment to prevention and early care. Indeed, there can now be a perverse incentive for the primary care provider to refer patients early and often to the higher levels of care, so that money allocated for primary care can be saved.

How will a 'capitation' fee model operate to efficiency? Ideally, care should be provided by a provider network that links several primary care providers with secondary and tertiary care hospitals. The money is paid to the network 'per capita', for each individual person to be covered. If primary care is efficient, need for secondary and tertiary care is reduced and the network saves money. To prevent under-provision or rationing of care (avoidance of referral to advanced care even when needed), standard management guidelines are to be developed and intermittent technical audits conducted. Overall, such a system is likely to result in better health outcomes and financial savings for the health system. By abandoning this linkage, NHP 2017 dissipates the advantage of the 'capitation' model in primary care while remaining vulnerable to the high costs of provider-induced care at secondary and tertiary levels.

Single Payer System

The policy has a stated intent to move to a 'single payer system' by merging central- and state-funded health insurance schemes. This can certainly help extend coverage through an expanded resource pool and provide the purchaser (the government) greater negotiating leverage in determining the pricing of procured services through the power of monopsony. How far this can be achieved in a multi-party federal polity, where government-funded health financing schemes carry political branding, remains to be seen. Will the central government set an example by merging the central government health scheme, which covers its own employees, with other centrally funded health insurance schemes?

The proposal to scrap 'user fee' and provide cashless service at the point of delivery is welcome. However, will this pre-paid mechanism be principally driven by tax revenue-funded direct healthcare provisioning or by health insurance-mediated payment? The preference indicated by the policy for the insurance route may run counter to the goal of providing appropriate care with optimal use of public financing. These questions have not been fully answered by the National Health Protection Mission, which emerged under the label of Ayushman Bharat in 2018.

Role of the Private Sector

The organised private sector has grown in presence and influence over the past four decades, capturing large segments of tertiary and secondary care from the under-resourced public sector. At the same time, individual primary care providers—qualified and unqualified—are scattered widely across India in an unorganised, even unregistered manner. The NHP proposes to access the services of the private sector to supplement those provided by the public sector, through empanelment and strategic purchasing. Thereby, the NHP represents a muting of the commitment to promote the public sector's pre-eminence and sends a clear call to the private sector to accept the government's invitation to partner in the delivery of services. Whether the private sector's role will be complementary, in the nature of gap filling, or if it will progressively displace the public sector will depend on the models of UHC that the centre and states adopt. The need to develop robust regulatory systems that can ensure cost and quality controls is all the more essential with the direction the NHP is taking for engaging the private sector.

Human Resources for Health

The aspirations articulated by the NHP can only be realised if there is a numerically adequate, socially motivated, multi-layered, multidisciplinary health workforce in place to deliver the intended services. Here, India faces a major challenge with shortages across the board among the various categories of healthcare providers, aggravated by mal-distribution across the states and an urban–rural mismatch.

Expanded institutional capacity, and new courses and cadres are proposed to overcome the shortages of skilled human resources in the health system. The NHP proposes to open more medical colleges, including new colleges attached to upgraded district hospitals. Training and deployment of mid-level healthcare providers has been proposed through nursing practitioners, bridge courses for AYUSH graduates and allied health professionals. A variety of specialised nursing and paramedical courses are proposed, even as ASHAs can career-track to become Auxiliary Nurse Midwives (ANMs). Recognising the deficiency of public health and managerial expertise in the health system, the NHP proposes to create Public Health Management Cadres in every state. Many of these proposals can infuse much-needed human resources to raise the level of health system performance, but speed is needed in implementing them.

Mainstreaming of AYUSH

A welcome feature of the NHP is the recognition given to the traditional systems of healthcare and healing, and the avowed intent to mainstream them into public sector health services at all levels. However, this commitment will be undermined by the expediency with which AYUSH professionals are being steered into allopathic practice through 'bridge courses' that will help to fill gaps in primary healthcare locations where allopathic doctors are not in place. Unless AYUSH professionals are supported in applying the knowledge and skills they have acquired in their own disciplinary education, their contribution to healthcare will be ineffective. They can and should, however, be trained in public health and inducted into the proposed Public Health Management cadres.

Disease Control Programmes

Health transition in India has brought NCDs and mental health disorders to the fore. However, the challenge of infectious and nutritional diseases still remains a public health priority, along with the need to accelerate declines in maternal and child mortality. The NHP addresses all of these in a wide-ranging array of vertical disease control programmes, but their intended operational integration on a health system platform, ideally through an expanded NHM, is not clearly described.

A variety of disease control measures and targets have been proposed to tackle challenges ranging from HIV-TB co-infection to trauma care and screening for hypertension, diabetes and common cancers (oral, cervical and breast). Tobacco control continues to be accorded high priority in the NHP, despite recent political opposition from powerful interests allied with the tobacco industry. The rising burden of NCDs, mental illness and injuries has been appropriately recognised for programmatic response.

Drugs, Diagnostics and Technologies

The policy proposes to provide essential drugs and diagnostics free of cost at public facilities. Depending on the extent to which these services are accessible, substantial early impact on out-of-pocket health expenditure is possible, relieving the financial burden on individuals. Wider market availability of generic drugs is promised through an expanded network of Jan Aushadi stores.

Social and Environmental Determinants of Health

While according high priority to water, sanitation and nutrition, the NHP brings up the problem of air pollution for the first time as a major health challenge. Both indoor and outdoor air pollution are listed as health threats that warrant a multi-sectoral response. It is proposed to build analytic capacity for health impact assessment of policies and programmes that affect health. With such modelled and measured assessments, based on robust research methodology, the health department would no longer be the passive recipient and *post-facto* responder of adverse effects resulting from health-eroding policies and programmes in other sectors, but can proactively influence those policies to be sensitive and responsive to public health needs and concerns.

Regulatory Systems

The Clinical Establishments Act, not adopted by many states so far, is sought to be uniformly enacted and implemented across the country. A National Healthcare Standards Organisation is proposed to be established to develop evidence-based standard management guidelines. A National Health Information Network also would be established by 2025. A National Digital Health Authority would be set up to develop, deploy and regulate digital health across the continuum of care. While these are welcome, the autonomy, transparency and effectiveness of the regulatory bodies need to be watched as they emerge and evolve. Further, the regulation of pharmaceutical products and their pricing, and also the reform and regulation of health professional education are still not adequately addressed.

NHP 2017 provides a matrix for improving access to health services. The priority accorded to primary healthcare is appropriate, but will the needed investment in financial and human resources be made to provide comprehensive continuous primary healthcare, encompassing preventive, promotive, diagnostic, curative, rehabilitative and palliative services? There is a real danger that the drive to scale up service provisioning at secondary and tertiary care levels, via government-financed insurance schemes and strategic purchasing through fee for service payments, will disproportionately drain health budgets and leave primary healthcare further disadvantaged. This anomaly will be aggravated by the disconnect between primary healthcare, which has to be delivered by the National Health Mission, and the health insurance schemes that will be managing the delivery of secondary and tertiary care. How the policy will address these contradictions, as it moves to implementation, remains to be seen.

References

Ministry of Health and Family Welfare, Government of India. 2003. 'National Health Policy'.

———. 2015. 'Draft National Health Policy 2015'.

———. 2017. 'National Health Policy 2017'. New Delhi. Available at http://cdsco.nic.in/writereaddata/National-Health-Policy.pdf (accessed 22 February 2019).

United Nations Development Programme. 2015. 'Sustainable Development Goals (SDGs)'.

World Health Organization. 2015. 'Millennium Development Goals (MDGs)'.

eight

Ayushman Bharat

> The new National Health Protection Scheme has the potential not only to improve health, but to help lift people out of poverty. The reforms which India is embarking on are bold, and they must be.
>
> Tedros Adhanom Ghebreyesus, 2018 (Sharma 2018)

Budget 2018 Brings a Blockbuster

Although the spotlight was turned on to Ayushman Bharat as a major new initiative in 2018, the narrative actually commenced two years earlier. The Union Finance Minister announced, in his budget speech of 2016, the government's intent to launch new schemes to improve the outreach of health services and provide the poor with financial protection for healthcare (Ministry of Finance 2016). A proposal to set up Health and Wellness Centres (HWCs) at the level of the health sub-centre was intended to improve rural primary healthcare. Revamping the pre-existing RSBY into a National Health Protection Scheme (NHPS) was also announced. The RSBY's annual coverage cap of Rs 30,000 per family was raised to Rs 1,00,000 to provide higher cost coverage for hospitalised care of the informal workers and other vulnerable groups registered in the earlier scheme.

Despite the prominent mention of these initiatives in the union budget of 2016, there was public silence on these two initiatives for the next two years. Clearly, there was no consensus within the government on how to configure and operate these schemes. In the budget of 2017, no mention was made of the NHPS and the nomenclature of the RSBY was maintained in the allocations to the health ministry. The health ministry's proposal to create a National Health Agency (NHA) and State Health Agencies (SHAs) to administer this scheme stalled as a result.

However, both HWCs and NHPS were again unveiled, with great prominence, in the union budget of 2018. Coupled under the evocative title of Ayushman Bharat (Long Life to India), the two initiatives covered services at different levels of healthcare, to improve coverage and extend financial protection (Ministry of Finance 2018). Positioned in this manner, the two initiatives were perceived by the media and public to be imaginative new initiatives that could transform healthcare. The NHPS, in particular, became headline news in both Indian and foreign media, being labelled quickly as Modicare or Namocare after the Prime Minister, who was credited as its architect. The scheme won plaudits from the Director General of the WHO and the editor of *Lancet*, a leading medical journal, as a major step towards universal health coverage (Horton 2018; Sharma 2018).

The scheme underwent several name changes from the time of its fresh unveiling in February 2018 to its launch in September 2018. It was initially relabelled as a scheme, the Pradhan Mantri Rashtriya Swasthya Suraksha Yojana. Later on, it was renamed as a mission to accord it a higher priority in the policy arena (the National Health Protection Mission). The name was then popularised as the Pradhan Mantri Jan Arogya Yojana (PMJAY), using Hindi nomenclature.

Comprehensive Primary Health Care (CPHC)

Ayushman Bharat proposes to convert 1,50,000 primary health sub-centres into HWCs. These transformed centres can be potential game changers in primary care, if properly configured, staffed, funded, mandated and managed. They will be redesigned to provide a wide range of essential primary health services close to home and will have both facility-based and community outreach services (National Health Portal 2019). As the frontline outposts of comprehensive primary healthcare, they are expected to deliver these services through a team of non-physician healthcare providers.

The CPHC builds upon the platform established by the NRHM, in aiming to strengthen primary health service delivery. While the NRHM was focussed on maternal and child health services, the NHP of 2017 calls for the NHM to become the vehicle for comprehensive, continuous primary care. This requires expansion of services to cover hitherto unattended areas like NCDs and mental health disorders. Ultimately, the NHM has to become the unifying platform for primary health services related to maternal and child health, communicable and non-communicable diseases, mental health and common disorders of eye, ear, nose and joints, apart from advancing health promotion efforts in the community. Surprisingly, dental care has remained outside the ambit of this comprehensive care palette, despite the high level of oral and dental health needs in the many sections of the community, from the poor to the elderly.

For future planning, India could draw a lesson from the Family Health Teams of Brazil, each of which has a physician, a nurse and six community health workers and looks after 3,000–4,000 people. Each community health worker serves a maximum of 150 households. The core team is also supported by a co-located dental team. Each group of four or five family health teams also receives specialist support from psychologists, community pharmacists and physiotherapists (Macinko and Harris 2015). Paucity of doctors and allied health professionals limits India's capacity to readily adopt and implement such a programme, but the future development of our health system, with higher investments in scaling up our health workforce, should aim for similar family health teams. Well-trained nurse practitioners or other mid-level healthcare providers will be able to meet many healthcare needs at the sub-centre level even if doctors are not presently part of the team. However, a fully developed team should aim to position doctors at least for intermittent support as needed.

Continuity of care requires that long-term care of chronic diseases is enabled through efficient follow-up at the primary care level, which has reliable bi-directional referral and return linkages with advanced care at the secondary and tertiary levels. Though primary care has even previously had elements of continuous care underlying antenatal follow-up visits and monitored treatment of tuberculosis and HIV-AIDS, services had been mostly configured for acute, episodic care. With the growing need to provide long-term care for chronic conditions like hypertension, diabetes and mental health disorders, primary care services have to be reconfigured to assure continuity of care. Health promotion, through community-level health education and individual counselling at the healthcare facility level, is an important activity that has so far been largely neglected in primary care. Just as healthy diets, regular physical activity and tobacco avoidance must be advocated in communities, missed opportunities for assisting tobacco cessation must be minimised in primary healthcare facilities.

The proposal to transform sub-centres into HWCs gives shape to comprehensive primary care at the frontline and enables continuity of care. It also brings basic health services closer to the homes of people in rural areas. Apart from facility-based care, community outreach would also strengthen health promotion and disease prevention. Augmented by induction of non-physician healthcare providers such as nurse practitioners, in addition to the existing staff, the HWC is also mandated to provide essential drugs and basic diagnostics free of cost. Various vertical disease control programmes will find convergence at this delivery point. With appropriate use of information technology, HWCs can generate real-time data for disaggregated estimates and monitoring of various health indicators. Judicious use of telemedicine and mobile phone technologies can help improve the delivery of healthcare at HWCs, through engagement of distant doctors.

It has been proposed that each HWC will serve 5,000 persons. A Primary Health Centre (PHC) will have six such HWCs connected to it. Apart from the nurse practitioner, it is expected to have two multi-purpose health workers (one female and one male). The HWC will combine a wide range of basic healthcare functions, along with wellness promotion through integration of AYUSH, promotion of healthy diets, regular physical activity, yoga, advocacy of tobacco avoidance and substance abuse, vector control, sanitation, hygiene and clean water programmes.

While the activation of HWCs is welcome, efforts to strengthen primary health services must extend also to primary and community health centres. The budgetary allocation to the NHM in 2018 and 2019 does not reflect the commitment to boost rural primary healthcare to the level needed. It is also disappointing to see that the Urban Health Mission component of the NHM has been virtually ignored in these budgets. Urban primary healthcare has been far too long neglected in both design and delivery. With increasing rural to urban migration, and the growth of urban slums and low-income communities, primary health services in cities and town acquires great urgency. HWCs will be needed for urban populations, too. The sum of Rs 1,200 crore allotted for HWCs will need to be substantially increased as the effort is scaled up.

The major challenge for developing fully functional HWCs is the shortage of human resources. While PHCs have suffered from non-availability of doctors, HWCs will be staffed by non-physician healthcare providers only. However, there is a need to create mid-level healthcare providers like nurse practitioners and community health assistants who have gone through a three-year degree programme, which is tailored to primary healthcare needs. The proposal to deploy AYUSH graduates (trained in traditional systems of medicine), with a bridge course orientation to allopathic medicine, is controversial and has met with resistance from the Indian Medical Association (Medical Dialogues 2018). Ideally, AYUSH practitioners should be placed in HWCs to provide expertise in the traditional systems of healing and health promotion wherein they have been trained (Reddy 2018). Apart from two Auxiliary Nurse Midwives, a male multi-purpose worker also would be needed to support the mid-level provider to ensure the delivery of intended services by the HWC. A laboratory-technician-cum-drug-dispenser would also be needed. Creating the human resource pool needed for HWCs will require a major effort, but will also result in job creation for many young people. Most importantly, it will build the defences of health and portals of healthcare close to the community.

National Health Protection Mission (PMJAY)

The PMJAY builds on the experience and lessons of the RSBY. While the poor gained increased access to secondary healthcare through the RSBY, the coverage was limited to Rs 30,000 annually per family. It had to compete in some states with state-funded health insurance schemes, which offered annual coverage variably capped between Rs 1,00,000 to Rs 3,30,000 per family. More importantly, it failed to provide financial protection against out-of-pocket health expenditure, catastrophic expenditure or healthcare-induced impoverishment. The ability to engage both public and private providers and the creation of strong information technology platforms have been gains from the RSBY experience. However, disconnect with primary care has minimised the impact of these central and state health insurance schemes on population health indicators.

The PMJAY offers Rs 5,00,000 cover per annum for 100 million poor and vulnerable families, to support hospitalised care. This covers approximately 500 million beneficiaries or 40 per cent of the population. They are to be identified on the basis of the Socio Economic and Caste Census (SECC), last conducted in 2011 (Ministry of Rural Development n.d.). The scheme does not call for premium-paid enrolment by the beneficiaries, who will instead be identified by the SECC and registered as eligibles. Since this is a fully government paid programme, it is being described as an 'assurance' programme, rather than an 'insurance' programme.

The PMJAY was initially proposed to be administered by an NHA, which will link to its state-level counterparts, the SHAs. Under the scheme, service would be provided by empanelled public and private hospitals at secondary and tertiary care levels. All public facilities, from the Community Health Centre to the district and medical college hospitals, would be automatically empanelled. Private hospitals would be empanelled based on defined criteria and would be linked to specific service packages (for example, paediatrics, gynaecology, cardiology, neurosurgery, cancer, etc.). The services would be cashless at the point of delivery. The SHA will be responsible for hospital empanelment, beneficiary identification, awareness generation among the beneficiaries, grievance redressal, fraud prevention, analytics and overall administration of the scheme within the state. In January 2019, the NHA and SHA were renamed as National Health Authority and State Heath Authority (instead of agencies), conferring more executive powers (Ghosh 2019).

The substantial raise in the proposed level of cost coverage, from the per family cap of Rs 30,000 per year in RSBY, will probably reduce the levels of catastrophic health expenditure, but will not impact regular out-of-pocket expenditure, since outpatient care is not covered. HWCs and other primary care strengthening efforts should ideally provide relief in that area. Efficient primary care services will also be required to reduce the need for secondary and tertiary care services and act as a prudent gatekeeper for referral to advanced care. In the absence of effective primary health services, the uncontrolled demand for services under the PMJAY will drain the health budget and, in turn, reduce the funds available for primary care and public-sector hospital strengthening.

Only Rs 2,000 crore were allotted for the PMJAY in the budget of 2018, as the scheme was scheduled for launch only in the latter half of the year. As utilisation rates rise with greater beneficiary awareness, the financing needs of the PMJAY will rise even further. The funding requirement would rise five to 10-fold when the PMJAY becomes fully operational in 2019. The overall central government allocation to Ayushman Bharat in the interim budget of 2019 is Rs 6,400 crore for the financial year 2019–20. This is likely to fall short of the requirements (Jaswal 2019). State governments are expected to contribute 40 per cent of the cost and will be encouraged to merge state-funded health insurance schemes with the PMJAY. Apart from expanding the resource pool and widening the 'risk pool' of the population to be covered, such a merger will also ensure portability of coverage to persons who move across state borders. However, this calls for consensus across different political parties governing across the country.

Alignment with State Schemes

Twenty states initially agreed to partner with the PMJAY but others have expressed their reservations. These relate to the proportion of beneficiaries covered, the process for identifying them and alignment with pre-existing state government-funded schemes. Odisha, for example, has launched the Biju Swasthya Kalyana Yojana, merging pre-existing financing schemes and providing 'universal' coverage in its inclusivity. This scheme too proposes Rs 5,00,000 cover per family, mostly for tertiary care, and will provide this protection to 70 per cent of the families in the state. This has been further enhanced to Rs 7,00,000 for women, to pay for their wide-ranging healthcare needs. Free health services at all public facilities up to the level of the district hospital have been assured, independent of this scheme, with all user charges waived. A drop-back assistance grant of Rs 500 would be provided to pregnant women and sick infants for return travel home (Patnaik 2018).

States with pre-existing schemes are wrestling with the process for reconciling their schemes, with a larger number or differently identified beneficiaries than in the PMJAY, with the new central scheme. Maharashtra and Rajasthan are among the states experiencing this unease. In Maharashtra, the currently operating Mahatma Jyotiba Phule Jan Arogya Yojana provides cover up to Rs 2,00,000 to 88 per cent of the families in the state. There is apprehension of a backlash if several of the present beneficiaries are excluded. Rajasthan has an existing 'health card' that is used to identify beneficiaries and is also contractually tied to an insurance company till 2019. The state's Bhamashah Swasthya Bima Yojana presently provides cashless health services to 450 million persons with a ceiling of Rs 3,30,000 (Ghosh 2018). As 2019 began, the states of Chhattisgarh and West Bengal have announced their intent to withdraw from the programme, replacing it with state-specific designs (Sharma 2019).

These problems of centre–state disconnect can be addressed only if the principle of universal free coverage is accepted for an identified set of services and cost coverage, through social protection schemes like the PMJAY, and is initially provided for other services only to the poor, the near-poor and other vulnerable sections of society. This pattern has to be uniform across the country. State and central resources have to be pooled together to ensure the maximum health and protection that can be obtained from the available resources. As both the centre and the states commit more resources to health, the level of protection and the number of beneficiaries covered can increase. This must be done always keeping in mind that primary care and secondary care up to the district hospital level must be accorded the highest priority and that preferential funding for tertiary care will be counterproductive.

A welcome feature of 2018 is the springing of competitive offerings by central and state governments that are committing public finance to support access to healthcare through new schemes, even though this rush does carry the danger of poor prioritisation. While these schemes will not amount to UHC, and by themselves will not assure the delivery of quality services, the attention given to health as part of the emerging political agenda bodes well for advancing efforts towards UHC. Much of this interest has arisen in the pre-election year. How far this enthusiastic espousal of public financing will remain at a high pitch after the elections of 2019, and whether the central and state budgets from now on provide for progressive increases in the allocations to health, remains to be seen. It will be good for the health of the nation if there is a broad consensus across all political parties to accord high priority to health and ensure policy continuity for advancing towards UHC.

Strategic Purchasing of Services

Strategic purchasing is the process by which the PMJAY proposes to judiciously purchase services from empanelled public and private hospitals. This requires a careful choice of the diseases, tests and treatments to be covered, development and adoption of evidence-based standard clinical management guidelines, setting and monitoring of cost and quality standards, and measurement of health outcomes. Fraud detection and grievance redressal mechanisms, too, need to be developed. Public awareness of the benefits offered under the PMJAY ('insurance literacy') must be promoted to increase registration and guide appropriate utilisation. If all of these safeguards are not in place, there will be danger of induced demand (unnecessary tests and treatments) escalating the costs of care provided through the PMJAY.

The process of strategic purchasing should not be to the disadvantage of public hospitals. Private hospitals say that government hospitals have the comparative advantage of government land and budgetary funding. However, the for-profit private hospitals have high levels of private investment, apart from receiving several government concessions in pricing of land and equipment. They are much better positioned to compete in the area of tertiary care and even in some areas of secondary care. A private hospital can attract more private investment from India and abroad, which a public hospital cannot. A private hospital can also take a bank loan to purchase state-of-the-art equipment, which a public hospital is not permitted to. Strategic purchasing will not fulfil its function if public hospitals are hobbled and asked to race with well-bred private hospitals. Therefore, governments must accord high priority to strengthening public hospitals and support them during the strategic purchasing process. Otherwise, the progressive decline of public-sector hospitals and excessive dependence on public-sector hospitals can result in the danger of private hospital cartels emerging to set high package rates for publicly funded service provision.

While the PMJAY and the state-level government schemes will raise the demand for hospital services, the supply side of service provision will be found wanting in many states. This is due to poor infrastructure and lack of required personnel in the public sector and the limited presence of organised private-sector hospitals in small and medium-sized towns. The government is offering a bouquet of financial incentives to the private sector to develop new hospitals in tier-2 and tier-3 cities. These include: land allotment; Viability Gap Funding (VGF) up to 40 per cent of the total cost of the project; gap funding up to 50 per cent of tax on capital cost; facilitation of permissions and clearances through special window with timelines and compulsory empanelment of the hospitals for the PMJAY and other government schemes. The government has also offered to restore the status of the 'hospital as an industry' for getting the benefit of VGF (Press Information Bureau 2019).

While the sense of urgency displayed by the government in trying to strengthen service provision by bridging the supply side gaps is welcome, the degree of tilt towards the private sector is a matter of concern. Will the private sector expand to fill all gaps across the country or cherry pick lucrative locations? Will the lax regulatory framework permit the private hospitals to milk the PMJAY scheme through induced demand for inappropriate care? Will the growing dependence on the private sector weaken the government's negotiating power on service package prices? What happens to the land and public investment if the private hospital withdraws from the PMJAY after a couple of years citing unattractive payment rates? Or if it markedly restricts the number of admissions under the PMJAY? These are points to ponder as the contracts are framed.

Of even greater concern is, should this public financing go instead, wholly or substantially, to expanding and strengthening public healthcare facilities such as district and sub-district hospitals? Will the fund flow to private sector, both for setting up hospitals and paying for PMJAY patients at negotiated rates, progressively reduce the funding needed to strengthen primary healthcare and district hospitals? Will urban primary healthcare become the main victim of the government's largesse to the private sector? These issues are likely to be vigorously debated as the PMJAY rolls on.

Administering the PMJAY

The NHA and state-level SHAs will oversee the design and implementation of the PMJAY. The administration of the PMJAY will be through a trust or an insurance company (Ahuja 2018). The choice of the intermediary will be left to the state governments. A trust, established by the government, has greater public accountability and less overheads (Reddy 2018). An insurance company comes with prior expertise in strategic purchasing and payments, but has more expensive overheads and is likely to demand higher premiums as the utilisation rates go up. In either case, it is the government that pays the premiums. While this differs from an individually purchased insurance scheme, the principle of 'risk pooling' is common. In a large risk pool, the healthy cross-subsidise the sick in any given year, keeping the premiums down. Though the PMJAY is a targeted programme for the poor and vulnerable families, financed from tax revenues of the government, an opportunity can potentially be provided for the non-poor also to buy into this scheme by paying the premiums set for the PMJAY. Such a mechanism will expand the risk pool, enhancing the degree of cross-subsidy, and provide those presently outside the ambit of PMJAY to benefit from the pre-paid services and financial protection offered by the scheme.

The entitlements promised by the PMJAY can only be delivered if adequate number of skilled doctors and allied health professionals are available to provide secondary and tertiary care. The need for producing more basic doctors and specialists was recognised in the NHP, as also the necessity of strengthening district hospitals. The budget of 2018 proposed to start 24 new medical colleges, with attachment to upgraded district hospitals. A medical college has been envisaged for every three parliamentary constituencies. This too calls for higher levels of public financing, as private-sector investment in medical colleges has mostly been limited to a few states. The overall increase in the health budget, however, was only 2.8 per cent over the revised estimates for the previous year's allocation. Allocation for establishment of new medical colleges has been reduced by 12.5 per cent. Unless the budgets from now on show a substantial year-on-year increase, the NHP target for public financing of 2.5 per cent of GDP by 2025 is unlikely to be attained.

How will Primary Healthcare and the PMJAY Connect?

While there is an avowed intent to seamlessly connect the programmes for comprehensive primary healthcare with secondary and tertiary care provision under the PMJAY, there is an administrative divide which raises concerns about this happening in reality. HWCs and comprehensive primary healthcare are under the purview of the NHM, steered by the central and state health ministries. The PMJAY is under autonomous NHA and SHAs. Primary healthcare has not been assigned a gatekeeper function for entry to the PMJAY. Given the current weakness of primary healthcare, it may be unrealistic to do so immediately. However, sooner than later, primary care has to bi-directionally connect to secondary- and tertiary-care facilities in a well-designed and efficiently managed pathway. Administrative and operational disconnects between the NHM and the PMJAY can spell danger to the objectives of Ayushman Bharat. There are also overlapping issues of healthcare financing, which need to be resolved. Will the PMJAY compete with, or even undermine, Janani Suraksha Yojana, which already has a health-financing programme, which provides pregnant women with care that extends from home to hospital? Caesarean sections, for example, could become an area of competition with unintended consequences.

Moving Health to the Market?

One of the disturbing features of the discourse around the PMJAY is the enthusiasm around the growth that the programme would stimulate in the private healthcare and private health insurance enterprises. While the growth of private healthcare facilities is a progressive phenomenon, the idea that this mission will depend a great deal on that growth for its success weighs against a balanced approach to UHC. Signals of such thinking emerge from early statements from the lead administrator of Ayushman Bharat. He is reported to have said that demand for services is likely to explode, with the expansion of affordable healthcare, 'with 5 million more procedures' in the country and the need for '35 million more hospital beds'. When asked how the health sector would cope, he is reported to have averred that the 'market will do that' (Doshi 2018). The faith placed in private-sector-led delivery of the PMJAY has subsequently been reiterated by policymakers and administrators (Kant and Bhushan 2018). The belief that the private sector would equitably and ethically fill all gaps in health services by applying market principles, while accessing public funding, is not merely overoptimistic. It may be delusory.

When most leading economists in the world agree that health represents an area of 'market failure', calling for government interventions and public-sector provisioning, to project the PMJAY as a launch pad for market-driven healthcare runs counter to global experience. Private-sector engagement in delivering the PMJAY, and ultimately UHC, is surely needed, but the government must not let this mission become the prime exemplar of market failure in delivering appropriate healthcare or creating an assembly line for more procedures than needed. While it is the responsibility of a caring government to provide hospitalised care to those who need it, the vision should not become constricted to focus only on that segment ignoring primary care and health promotion.

Addressing the other Determinants of Health

The budget of 2018 also addressed some of the social and environmental determinants of health. Rupees six hundred crore were allocated to provide financial support to patients of tuberculosis to improve their nutrition, through a monthly stipend of rupees five hundred. This will help to boost their immunity and improve treatment results. The sanitation component of the Swachh Bharat mission was funded for scale-up through the construction of more toilets, to reduce the health hazards of open defecation. Air pollution, the second most important cause of ill health in India according to a recent estimate, was intended to be addressed through interventions aimed at both ambient and indoor air pollution (Air Pollution Collaborators 2019). Delhi's neighbouring states were to be provided financial support for promoting in-situ disposal of crop waste by non-burning methods. The Ujjwala scheme was to be expanded to provide cooking gas connections to more poor women, to help them and their young children escape the kitchen's curse of air pollution from combustion of solid biomass fuels. Risks of respiratory diseases, cardiovascular disorders, cancers, childhood asthma and respiratory infections, and even diabetes, will be reduced through control of air pollution.

While these are good initiatives to promote or protect health through actions in other sectors, many well-coordinated multi-sectoral programmes would be required to influence the social and environmental determinants of health at the population and community levels. Primary Health Care offers a good platform for inter-sectoral convergence and community mobilisation, while providing a window for examining the ground-level impact of population-level policy interventions. Ayushman Bharat should enable HWCs to play this role by building the capacity of all health personnel engaged in delivering primary health services for catalysing and coordinating multi-sectoral action.

Judging by the media attention and the political pitch, the union budget of 2018 placed health in the centre-stage of public discourse. However, the success of the ambitious initiatives that have been proposed depends on a sizeable and progressive increase in financial resources allocated to health in both central and state budgets from now on and a concerted effort to build wide-ranging capacity in the health system. The NHP 2017 calls on states to increase their health budgets to exceed 8 per cent of their total budgets by 2020. It is imperative that they do so, even as the central government keeps its promise of raising its share of public financing for health. Investment in a multi-layered, multi-skilled workforce, capable of providing high quality services at all levels of care, is essential. These must be coupled with strong regulatory and monitoring systems. Only when all of these progress in a concerted and timely manner will India advance with surety and success on the long path to universal health coverage.

References

Ahuja, R. 2018. 'National Health Protection Scheme: Choosing the Right Model for Implementation'. *Financial Express*, 29 March. Available at http://www.financialexpress.com/opinion/national-health-protection-scheme-choosing-the-right-model-for-implementation/1114431/ (accessed 24 December 2018).

Doshi, V. 2018. 'India is Rolling out a Health-care Plan for Half a Billion People. But are there Enough Doctors?' *The Washington Post*, 14 August. Available at https://www.washingtonpost.com/world/2018/08/14/india-is-rolling-out-healthcare-plan-half-billion-people-are-there-enough-doctors/?noredirect=on&utm_term=.5b4af5475a9c (accessed 24 December 2018).

Ghosh, A. 2018. 'NHPM: Two BJP States Wary, Maharashtra has no Funds after Loan Sop'. *The Indian Express*, 9 July.

———. 2019. 'National Health Authority Gets Cabinet Nod'. *Indian Express*, 3 January. Available at https://indianexpress.com/article/india/national-health-authority-gets-cabinet-nod-5520837/ (accessed 24 December 2018).

Horton, R. 2018. 'The New Politics of Health in India'. *Lancet* 392 (10151): 902.

India State-Level Disease Burden Initiative Air Pollution Collaborators. 2019. 'The Impact of Air Pollution on Deaths, Disease Burden, and Life Expectancy across the States of India: The Global Burden of Disease Study 2017'. *Lancet Planetary Health* 3 (1): e26–39.

Jaswal, M. 2019. 'Union Budget 2019: Government to Allocate Rs 6,400 Crore for Ayushman Bharat Scheme'. *Economic Times*, 1 February. Available at https://www.businesstoday.in/current/economy-politics/union-budget-2019-government-to-allocate-rs-6400-crore-for-ayushman-bharat-scheme/story/316068.html (accessed 1 February 2019).

Kant, A., and I. Bhushan. 2018. 'No Trade-offs in Healthcare'. *Indian Express*, 9 November. Available at https://indianexpress.com/article/opinion/columns/no-trade-offs-in-healthcare-pradhan-mantri-jan-arogya-yojana-health-care-5438330/ (accessed 17 December 2018).

Macinko, J., and M. Harris. 2015. 'Brazil's Family Health Strategy—Delivering Community-based Primary Care in a Universal Health System'. *New England Journal of Medicine* 372 (23): 2177–81.

Ministry of Finance, Government of India Budget 2016–17. 2016. 'Speech of Arun Jaitley'. Available at https://www.indiabudget.gov.in/ub2016-17/bs/bs.pdf (accessed 7 December 2018).

Ministry of Finance, Government of India Budget 2018–19. 2018. 'Speech of Arun Jaitley'. Available at https://www.indiabudget.gov.in/ub2018-19/bs/bs.pdf (accessed 7 December 2018).

Ministry of Rural Development, Government of India. n.d. 'Socioeconomic and Caste Census'. Available at https://secc.gov.in/reportlistContent (accessed 21 December 2018).

National Health Portal. 2019. 'Ayushman Bharat Yojana'. Available at https://www.nhp.gov.in/ayushman-bharat-yojana_pg (accessed 18 December 2018).

'NMC Bill: IMA Releases Point by Point Rebuttal to Health Ministry FAQs, Details Here'. *Medical Dialogues*. Available at https://medicaldialogues.in/nmc-bill-ima-releases-point-by-point-rebuttal-to-health-ministry-faqs/ (accessed 18 December 2018).

Patnaik, S. Biju. 2018. 'Swasthya Kalyan Yojana: 70 Lakh to be Covered, Odisha Starts Posting Health Scheme Letters'. *The Indian Express*, 16 August. Available at https://indianexpress.com/article/india/biju-swasthya-kalyan-yojana-70-lakh-to-be-covered-odisha-starts-posting-health-scheme-letters-naveen-patnaik-5309137/ (accessed 24 December 2018).

Press Information Bureau. 2019. 'Broad Guidelines for Private Investments in Setting up of Hospitals in Tier 2 and Tier 3 Cities Subsequent to PMJAY'. Available at http://pib.nic.in/newsite/PrintRelease.aspx?relid=187353 (accessed 24 December 2018).

Reddy, K. Srinath. 2018a. 'National Health Protection Scheme: Why Insurance can't Replace Primary Healthcare'. *Financial Express*, 9 February. Available at http://www.financialexpress.com/opinion/national-health-protection-scheme-why-insurance-cant-replace-primary-healthcare/1058904/ (accessed 24 December 2018).

———. 2018b. 'Remaking Medical Education'. *Deccan Herald*, 6 January. Available at https://www.deccanherald.com/content/652294/remaking-medical-education.html (accessed 21 December 2018).

Sharma, N. 2019. 'Chhattisgarh Govt to Pull out of Ayushman Bharat'. *The Economic Times*, 16 January. Available at https://economictimes.indiatimes.com/industry/healthcare/biotech/healthcare/chhattisgarh-govt-to-pull-out-of-ayushman-bharat/articleshow/67550227.cms (accessed 24 December 2018).

Sharma, Y. 2018. 'WHO Lauds National Health Protection Scheme, Ayushman Bharat'. *The Economic Times*, 15 March. Available at https://economictimes.indiatimes.com/industry/healthcare/biotech/healthcare/who-lauds-national-health-protection-scheme-ayushman-bharat/articleshow/63310006.cms?from=mdr (accessed 22 February 2019).

nine

The Way Forward

> A well ordered society would ensure that all individuals have the capability to be healthy and at a level that is commensurate with human dignity in the modern world, which is their right.
>
> Sridhar Venkatapuram, 2011

Just as the years 2005–07 have been landmarks in the odyssey of India's health policy, with the design and launch of the NRHM, the years 2017–18 have also been momentous for the attention they have brought to health policy. The new NHP was adopted in 2017. The year 2018 began with the budget announcing Ayushman Bharat and ended with the newly elected government of Chhattisgarh declaring that the state would not be bound by that scheme, but would follow a different path to UHC. What will 2019, a national election year, and the years beyond bring to health policy? While political power dynamics in central and state governments will undoubtedly influence the manner in which health policy will be shaped and implemented, an overarching commitment to primary healthcare-led UHC should set the coordinates for our journey into the future. Policymakers should aim and act towards implementing several important steps that will be outlined in this chapter.

Improve the Design and Delivery of Rural and Urban Primary Healthcare

The upgrading of sub-centres to HWCs is a good beginning but will require adequate investment in training, recruitment and well-distributed deployment of skilled and technology-enabled human resources, especially mid-level health workers like nurse practitioners and community health officers. Higher levels of primary healthcare, too, must be strengthened, from PHCs to community health centres, with attention to infrastructure, equipment, supplies, connectivity and, most important of all, adequate availability of health professionals of diverse categories. Well-designed incentive packages should be offered to make primary healthcare postings attractive to doctors, nurses and allied health professionals. Urban primary healthcare, long neglected, must be provided through easy-to-access neighbourhood health centres, principally served by technology-enabled nurse practitioners with intermittent physician visits.

Strengthen District Hospitals

District hospitals should be upgraded with investments in infrastructure, equipment and skilled human resources, to deliver hospitalised speciality care (secondary care), alongside outpatient care. In states which presently have low numbers of medical, nursing and allied health professional training colleges, upgraded district hospitals should become the clinical facility attached to new publicly financed health professional training institutions. These institutions should link with the district and sub-district health systems for undergraduate health professional training.

Scale up Human Resources for Health

The shortages in most categories of health service providers that debilitate our health system must be addressed with urgency. More medical, nursing and allied health professional institutions must be established in regions of the country, which now have very few. A National Commission for Human Resources in Health must be established to provide overarching direction to and ensure good governance of competency-based education that meets health system needs, matches contemporary standards and provides a platform for inter-professional education. Training programmes for medical specialists, nurse practitioners, advanced nursing, community health officers and public health professionals must be redesigned, standardised and scaled up. Human resource management needs to be improved, with cadre creations for clinical (medical, dental, nursing, allied health professionals) and public health functions.

To overcome the challenge of maldistribution of doctors, resulting in many underserved populations, a National Medical Service should be established with three levels of entry: (i) fresh medical graduates to be recruited to the NHM, as a common national pool, to serve a two-year short service commission in the primary healthcare system anywhere in the country; (ii) postgraduate specialist doctors to serve for three years in district hospitals, in a short service commission after receiving their degree; and (iii) permanent cadre of specialist and super-specialist doctors to be inducted into an all-India service akin to the Indian Administrative Service. They can link the various All-India Institutes of Medical Sciences and other central government institutions across the country and also be made available for state deputation. Central and state-level public health cadres, too, should be set up in accordance with the NHP 2017. All doctors in government service must be well paid, placed in full-time employment and made accountable for service delivery. Private practice should not divert government doctors from their duties and poor pay scales should not become a reason for seeking income elsewhere.

Provide Free Drugs and Diagnostics in all Public Healthcare Facilities

All drugs listed in the NLEM and, additionally, other drugs listed in the States' Lists of Essential Medicines should be provided free of cost in all public healthcare facilities. The cost should be shared between the centre and states. Pooled public procurement of quality assured generic drugs will ensure that the cost of procuring these drugs from Indian manufacturers is kept low. Such procurement should be undertaken by central and state-level procurement agencies modelled after the Tamil Nadu Medical Systems Corporation/Rajasthan processes. Private (especially not-for-profit) healthcare institutions accredited by government, as part of the UHC delivery network, should be provided an opportunity to benefit from the pooled procurement process of these autonomous agencies. This will help to offset the loss of income these private providers apprehend from their having to accept the cost controls built into the healthcare purchasing mechanism of UHC.

Domestic manufacture of drugs and devices must be encouraged by government policy. Bulk drug manufacture, too, must be supported by encouraging chemical industries which provide the basic ingredients. Drug testing and regulation must be strengthened through well-equipped central and state drug-testing laboratories and well-resourced regulatory agencies that have the required technical capacity and monitoring reach across the country.

While permitting multi-national drug companies to operate, price controls must be exercised on essential and lifesaving drugs. While respecting intellectual property, India should not surrender its right to invoke the compulsory licensing provision of the WTO when public health needs require it to do so. In this regard, international trade regulations must be carefully negotiated to avoid restrictions on India's ability to produce essential and lifesaving drugs.

The manufacture and regulation of devices require a different pathway from drugs. An autonomous body may be established for this purpose, drawing in technical expertise from several disciplines and utilising a governance structure which has representation from the departments of health, health research, biotechnology, science and technology, information technology, and industry. Incentives should be provided to domestic manufacturers for import substitution of commonly used devices and their consumables.

Diagnostic facilities should also be free at the point of care in all public healthcare facilities. Public financing, through tax-based budgetary allocations, should ensure this. Standard Management Guidelines, prepared by expert committees and approved by the government, will enable appropriate use of drugs and diagnostic tests.

Create Networks of Primary, Secondary and Tertiary Care Providers at District and State Levels

If easily accessible and efficient primary healthcare services must form the firm foundation of a district health system, it is also necessary that primary care is bi-directionally connected to higher levels of care, for appropriate referral and follow-up care on return. In a mixed health system, it becomes necessary to bring as many healthcare providers as possible into an integrated network of providers, which provides breadth at each level of care (primary, secondary and tertiary), and depth in the connectivity between these levels. Such a network should support the delivery of health services, which are offered in any programme of UHC. While including healthcare providers from public, private and voluntary sectors, the network must function under the overall direction of the public sector, which sets the terms and defines the deliverables. Such networks must be established at the level of each district, and function under the overall guidance of the district health officer. At the state level, the district networks could extend to partner other networks as per need (for example, for advanced healthcare, which is unavailable in a district, but exists in another). Schemes for UHC can contract these networks for provision of services to defined population groups under a capitation mode of payment, which covers all health services as needed at any level of care. Such a payment mode will incentivise the network to prioritise prevention and early care at the primary level to many, while making advanced care available to the fewer numbers who need it.

Increase Public Financing of Health and Move Towards a Single Payer System

For all of the above changes to happen, health budgets need to be increased at central and state levels. While this is often proclaimed as public policy, especially before elections, the rate of increase remains excruciatingly slow. A commitment must be made to increase public financing by at least 20 per cent each year for the next five years and must be earnestly implemented. The new state health policy of Kerala, released in January 2019, provides this commitment, stating that the government will aim at raising its expenditure on health from the current 0.6 per cent of Gross State Domestic Product to at least 5 per cent and strive to increase it by 1 per cent every year (Special Correspondent, *The Hindu* 2019). Even as public financing for health is increased, primary health services must be prioritised, with 70 per cent of the public financing committed and delivered to that vital component of health services.

For UHC to be truly delivered, with inclusivity of all population groups and portability across the whole country, all central and state government-funded healthcare financing schemes must be aligned to be complementary, if not fully merged. Ideally, a single payer system must emerge within five years.

To meet the objective of reducing out-of-pocket and catastrophic health expenditures, to whom and how much will be the cost coverage provided by the government? Primary healthcare, emergency health services, essential secondary care (such as for commonly required surgeries) and lifesaving tertiary care (for some clearly identified conditions) must be provided free to all. For other conditions (excluding conditions such as cosmetic surgery), poor and vulnerable sections must be provided free care.

If Ayushman Bharat continues in its present structure, what can be the mechanism by which a single payer system can emerge for UHC? Since the PMJAY scheme covers 40 per cent of the population, the remaining 60 per cent could be encouraged to join the scheme by paying income-graded premiums. These could include even employer-paid healthcare schemes. Even if a few rich opt out, a vast majority will be covered by one scheme. Co-branding of the centre and states will be needed for such a common pool to emerge. The recent scheme in Odisha, which offers free provision of primary and secondary services to all up to the district hospital level and provides cost coverage to 70 per cent of the state's population at the tertiary care level, may prove attractive to other states. All states, however, will have to grapple with the issue of ensuring portability of benefits to their registrants as they migrate for work or education. Every state also has to acknowledge the need to increase front-end spending on infrastructure, equipment, supplies and human resources to enhance the capacity of their health systems to deliver the promised entitlements. Even if this calls for higher initial investment, strengthening of primary healthcare and district hospitals will provide a population health dividend that will progressively reduce the costs of advanced care. If the governments prioritise hospitalised tertiary care instead, the health budgets will get increasingly sucked up by the escalating costs of such care. Since it is difficult to take U-turns, it is wise not to get locked into such schemes at the beginning of our journey towards UHC.

AYUSH and other Traditional Systems

India's rich indigenous health systems must be utilised to provide greater access to healthcare, both as an alternative to and complementary to allopathic medicine. Appropriate knowledge validation methods (beyond conventional clinical research methods) must be developed to identify how best these systems can be used for health promotion, disease prevention, clinical treatment and palliative care.

Improve Regulatory and Information Systems

If the quality of care provided under UHC has to meet and maintain acceptable standards, if the private sector is going to be invited to more extensively partner in government-financed schemes, if drugs and diagnostics are going to be provided at all public facilities through pooled public procurement, if competency-based health professional education and training programmes are going to be scaled up with unwavering commitment to integrity of accrediting bodies and if the health rights of citizens (especially patients) have to be protected, the existing regulatory systems will have to be revamped and new regulatory bodies will have to be created as may be needed. Attempting to transform the health system, while having weak or ineffective regulatory systems, is likely to result in serious distortions in access, quality and cost of health services.

Health management information systems also need to be redesigned to become capable of providing representative, disaggregated, real-time data on major health indicators, risk factors, disease outbreaks, health system performance (especially on access, costs of care and level of financial protection) and social determinants. India's strength in technology should be utilised to ensure this. A strong primary healthcare system will ensure that real-time data can be generated by technology-enabled frontline health workers, supplemented when needed by innovative methods such as crowd sourcing of reports during outbreaks.

Actively Involve the Community

It is both ethical and efficient to engage the public in the design, delivery, monitoring and evaluation of health programmes. 'Nothing about us without us!' was a slogan that emerged from the HIV-AIDS patient groups and persons with disabilities, but is relevant to the whole spectrum of health services. Citizens and patients have a right to have their voice heard and opinions taken into account in health policy matters that affect their lives and wellbeing. Even the implementation of health programmes will be more successful if people are engaged not only in the demand for services, but also in their delivery. Maternal and child health, nutrition, prevention of vector-borne diseases and anti-microbial resistance, tobacco control, alcohol and substance abuse, and mental health are among the examples of programmes where citizen groups and civil society organisations can actively contribute. The potential of women's self-help groups, youth groups and resident welfare associations needs to be tapped more. Citizen groups can also help to monitor and report on the performance of health programmes.

Adapting the models developed in Brazil and Thailand, Health Councils can be set up at village, municipality and district levels. State and national health assemblies should be organised annually to assess progress, recommend correctives and redefine priorities.

Create Momentum for Multi-sectoral Action on Social, Environmental and Commercial Determinants of Health

As the health of populations is profoundly influenced by determinants that are conventionally outside the remit of the health ministry and health system managers, health policy must proactively reach out to all health-relevant sectors to sensitise them to public health concerns and goals. Capacity for Health Impact Assessment must be developed to measure and model the current and prospective impact of policies and programmes in other sectors on health, through trans-disciplinary approaches. Based on such knowledge, a convincing social, economic and environmental case must be made by health ministries to inform and influence policies in other sectors and align them to the public health agenda.

While each of these steps requires distinctive, well-defined initiatives, they all need to be confluent and convergent to create health in the society, both through the health system and other sectors which impact health. For this, a vision needs to be developed that can lead to concerted actions that provide health assurance to the population. Such assurance should not be merely seen as cost coverage of services related to some elements of healthcare provided to some sections of the population or as a euphemism for health insurance. It should provide financial protection for all needed health services that any citizen avails through an adequately resourced and well-functioning health system. Such an assurance should also convey that public policy and governmental programmes will earnestly aim to influence the social determinants of health to promote healthy living conditions for all persons at all ages. Figure 9.1 portrays this vision in three concentric circles. The innermost is of financial protection for healthcare through health financing that is principally tax-based and supplemented by other sources. The second circle includes elements of the health system which are essential for delivering these funded services. These two circles together will provide UHC. The third circle adds social determinants, which act at the population and individual levels. Together, all the three circles constitute the holistic vision of health assurance (Reddy 2015).

To accomplish these necessary but challenging tasks that are critical to the transformation of India's health system, it is essential to build a political consensus around this agenda. Much of the past dissonance in health policy has arisen from non-consultative and often poorly informed priority setting. Without adequate centre–state consultations, consensus and coordination, any health policy reform will meet many road blocks. Consensus

Figure 9.1: Vision for Health Assurance

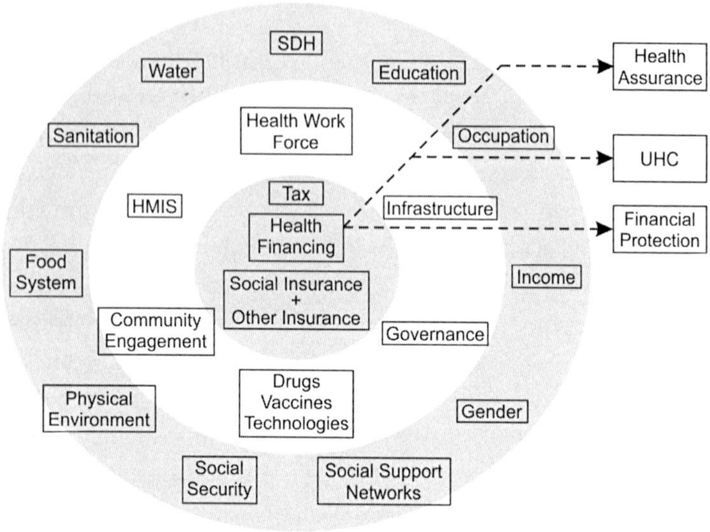

Source: Reddy 2015.

and common commitment, on adopting and implementing an agreed health agenda, are also needed among the many political parties that govern or oppose in different parts of the country. Will the leadership of all these political parties recognise that health is a precious human right and a vital area of human development that affects every Indian and should, therefore, be regarded as a high national priority? Will such a vision emerge from the collective wisdom of our political leaders? Will the citizens be able to nudge or even compel them to pay serious and sincere attention to health in the coming decade? The future of India's health—indeed, India's future itself—depends on the answers that will emerge in the coming years.

References

Reddy, K. Srinath. 2015. 'Health Assurance: Giving Shape to a Slogan'. *Current Medicine Research and Practice* 5 (1): 1–9.

Special Correspondent. 2019. 'Focus on Ensuring Quality Care in Public Health System in Kerala'. *The Hindu*, 25 January. Available at https://www.thehindu.com/news/national/kerala/focus-on-ensuring-affordable-care-in-public-health-system-in-kerala/article26081681.ece (accessed 25 January 2015).

Venkatapuram, S. 2011. *Health Justice: An Argument from the Capabilities Approach*. Cambridge: Polity Press.